KU-198-350

THE
HUMAN BODY

THE
HUMAN BODY

THE ESSENTIAL ILLUSTRATED REFERENCE

Vigué-Martín

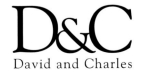

D&C
David and Charles

A DAVID & CHARLES BOOK

David & Charles is a subsidiary of F+W (UK) Ltd.,
an F+W Publications Inc. company

First published in the UK in 2005
Originally published as *Atlas del Cuerpo Humano* by GORG BLANC SL, Spain, 2004

Copyright © GORG BLANC 2004

All rights reserved. No part of this publication may be reproduced, stored in a retrieval
system, or transmitted, in any form or by any means, electronic or mechanical, by
photocopying, recording or otherwise, without prior permission in writing from the
publisher.

The author and publisher have made every effort to ensure the accuracy of the
information in this book and therefore cannot accept liability for any resulting injury,
damage or loss to persons or property however it may arise.

A catalogue record for this book is available from the British Library.

ISBN 0 7153 2258 3

Printed in Spain by Bigsa
for David & Charles
Brunel House   Newton Abbot   Devon

Visit our website at www.davidandcharles.co.uk

David & Charles books are available from all good bookshops; alternatively you can
contact our Orderline on (0)1626 334555 or write to us at FREEPOST EX2 110,
David & Charles Direct, Newton Abbot, TQ12 4ZZ (no stamp required UK mainland).

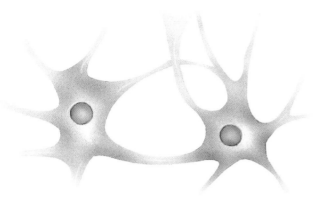

The human body is a formidable machine that carries out a series of functions: breathing, eating, reproduction, excretion of waste products and perceiving the outside world. Accomplishing each function requires the development of a specific system such as the respiratory, digestive, urinary and auditory systems. In turn, each system is composed of specific organs such as the heart, stomach, lungs and eyes.

Each organ and system depends on all the others to function correctly and contribute to the physiological balance that makes us human beings.

Like any machine, the body needs maintenance and care, both preventive and curative, to enable it to function without problems. Although it is very sophisticated and complex, knowledge of its composition and the way it functions is essential in maintaining health.

This book presents a systematic overview of the human body. It is divided into chapters, each of which describes a specific system. Each page consists of diagrammatic illustrations with relevant explanatory annotation, which together comprise a wealth of detail. The objective is not only to provide an attractive book, but also one that is capable of explaining any question the reader might have. Thus, as well as providing the practical application of an atlas, offers a wide-ranging amount of general and interesting information.

The characteristics of the atlas means it is suitable for a broad range of readers. The quality of the illustrations and their high level of detail, combined with the concise and precise textual explanations, make it useful for secondary students and teachers and for many professional groups – trainers, physiotherapists, gymnasts, sportsmen, homoeopaths, nurses, masseurs, and many others – as well as those beginning the study of medicine or the lay reader interested in health and in the care of their own body.

A special effort has been made to ensure the high quality of the book and to include information that may be lacking in comparable books.

We believe that *The Human Body* is an exciting new addition to the field of human anatomy.

We hope that as well as providing any information that the reader might seek, the book will help people care for their bodies and so improve their quality of life.

Jordi Vigué

SUMMARY

DIGESTIVE SYSTEM

THE RESPIRATORY SYSTEM

THE URINARY SYSTEM

THE REPRODUCTIVE SYSTEM

THE BLOOD

THE GLANDULAR SYSTEM

THE NERVOUS SYSTEM

THE SENSORY SYSTEM

THE STRUCTURE OF THE HUMAN BODY

atoms

Whatever form that matter adopts – solid, liquid or gas – it is always composed of tiny structural units called atoms, which are formed by a centre or nucleus containing the mass, and an orbital system containing gyrating electrons, particles with no mass and with a negative electric charge. The nucleus contains at least two other particles: neutrons, with no electric charge, and protons, with a positive electric charge. The equilibrium of the system is maintained by the balance between the positive electric charge (protons) and the negative charge (electrons). To date, 92 different electrons have been identified.

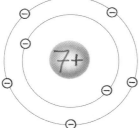

nitrogen

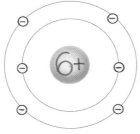

carbon

hydrogen

oxygen

elements

The grouping of atoms of the same type gives rise to elements. The four basic elements which form living matter are carbon, hydrogen, nitrogen and oxygen.

human body

The union and coordination of the different systems that form the complex structure that is the human body.

systems

The union of the different organs gives rise to the formation of different functional units that form the macroscopic structures of the human body, each of which has an overall function: nutrition, defence, support, regulation, etc.

compounds

The union of the different elements gives rise to the compounds, whose minimum expression is known as a molecule. An example is the water molecule, formed from two atoms of hydrogen and one of oxygen. The compounds that form living matter may be organic or inorganic, depending on whether they contain carbon atoms or not. The basic organic compounds are water, proteins, carbohydrates and fats, to which others, such as nucleic acids and steroids, are added.

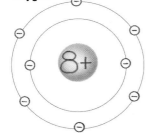

organs

The different tissues combine to form organs, structures that have a specific function or functions in the human body.

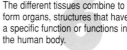

cells

The different compounds (water, carbohydrates, proteins, fats, nucleic acids, etc.) combine to form cells, which are living organisms with complicated mechanisms of nutrition, digestion, energy production, reproduction and, in many cases, movement. Many living organisms are single-celled, but the human body, the most complex living structure, is composed of more than 100 trillion cells.

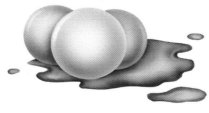

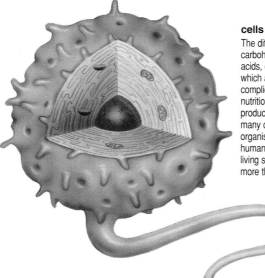

tissues

The cells of the human body combine to form more complicated anatomical elements. The main body tissues are squamous or pavement epithelial tissue (skin and mucous); secreting epithelial tissue (exocrine and endocrine glands); connective tissue (bones, cartilages, lungs, fatty tissue, etc.); muscular tissue; blood tissue (blood); lymph tissue (lymph nodes, bone marrow, etc.); and nervous tissue.

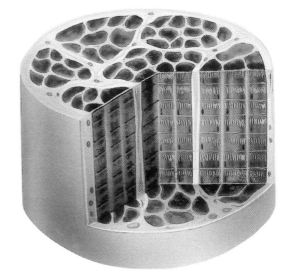

EXTERNAL ANATOMICAL FEATURES

▼ FEMALE ANTERIOR VIEW

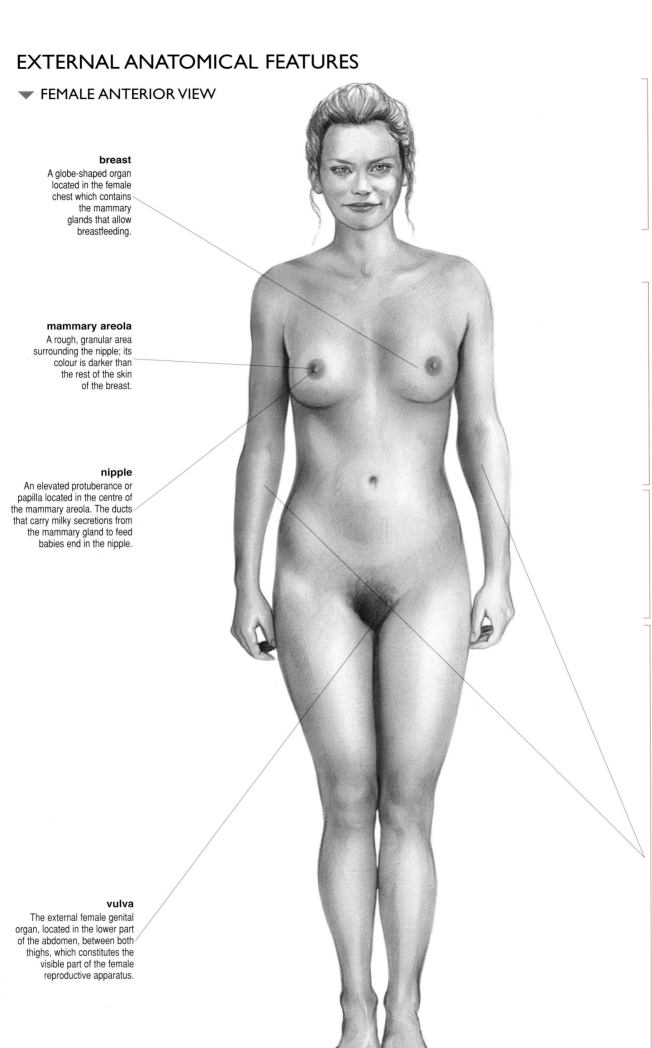

breast
A globe-shaped organ located in the female chest which contains the mammary glands that allow breastfeeding.

mammary areola
A rough, granular area surrounding the nipple; its colour is darker than the rest of the skin of the breast.

nipple
An elevated protuberance or papilla located in the centre of the mammary areola. The ducts that carry milky secretions from the mammary gland to feed babies end in the nipple.

vulva
The external female genital organ, located in the lower part of the abdomen, between both thighs, which constitutes the visible part of the female reproductive apparatus.

head
The upper part of the human body which contains the brain and most of the sense organs.

thorax
The area of the human body located between the head and the abdomen which contains the heart and lungs and where the upper extremities are inserted.

abdomen
The area of the human body located below the thorax, which extends from the waist to the groin. It is where the lower extremities are inserted and contains most of the alimentary canal, the spleen, the urinary system and the reproductive system.

limbs
The two upper and two lower limbs, known as the extremities, are inserted in the thorax and abdomen, respectively, and are composed of articulated portions. They are fundamental for movement, posture and bipedalism, and allow humans to move freely and accomplish complex manoeuvres, some exclusive to the human species.

9

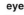

EXTERNAL ANATOMICAL FEATURES

▼ MALE ANTERIOR VIEW

ear
The fleshy, visible part of the hearing system, located at each side of the head. The ears collect sounds and channel them towards the acoustic duct.

nose
An appendix located in the centre of the face which connects the respiratory system with the exterior.

nipple
An elevated protuberance or papilla in the centre of the mammary areola.

waist
A fold or narrowing that separates the ribs from the hips.

navel
The residual scar left after tying off the foetal umbilical cord.

hip
A rim that is located on both sides of the abdomen below the waist and marks the hip bone.

groin
A lateral fold that ascends obliquely from the genital area and marks the area where the lower extremities are united with the abdomen.

fingernails
Accessory organs of the skin formed by hard, dense, keratinized cells that cover the posterior distal part of the fingers.

pubic region
A triangular area located in the lower part of the abdomen immediately above the genitals. In adults, it is usually covered in hair.

penis
The external male genital organ that has both urinary and reproductive functions.

scrotum
A saccular structure located between the thighs and behind the penis which contains the testicles or testes.

ankle
The joint that articulates the bones of the leg and the foot.

toes
Five small appendices located in the anterior zone of each foot.

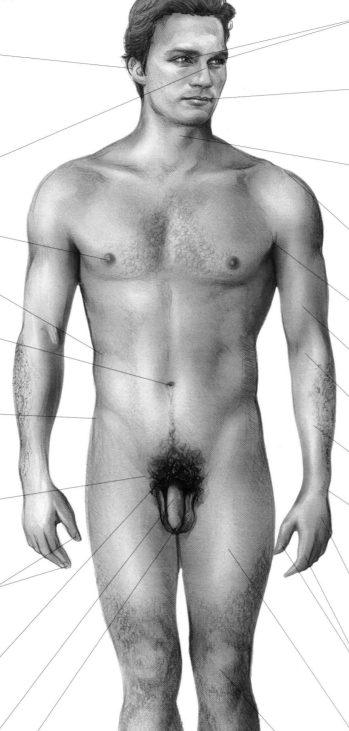

eye
The external organs of sight that are contained in the ocular or orbital cavities and protected by the eyelids.

mouth
An orifice located in the face that serves as the entrance to the digestive system and contains the external organs of the sense of taste.

neck
A tubular part of the body that unites the head with the thorax, and through which the digestive, respiratory and nervous systems pass.

shoulder
The area where the upper limb joins the thorax. Due to its powerful musculature, the shoulder usually has a rounded aspect.

armpit
A concave area located in the inferior angle of the union of the upper limb with the thorax. In adults, the armpit is usually covered with hair.

arm
The first portion of the upper limb that extends from the shoulder and the armpit to the elbow.

flexure of the elbow
The anterior face or flexure of the joint that articulates the arm and the forearm.

forearm
The portion of the upper extremity that extends from the elbow to the wrist.

wrist
The area that joins and articulates the bones of the forearm and the hand.

hand
The distal extremity of the upper limb that, thanks to the fingers, has great dexterity and contributes greatly to the distinctiveness of the human species.

fingers
The five distal extremities of each hand.

thigh
The upper part of the lower limb that extends from the groin to the knee.

knee
The middle area of the lower limbs where the thigh and leg are joined and articulated.

feet
The distal extremities of the lower limbs. They are essential for walking, posture and bipedalism.

EXTERNAL ANATOMICAL FEATURES

▼ MALE POSTERIOR VIEW

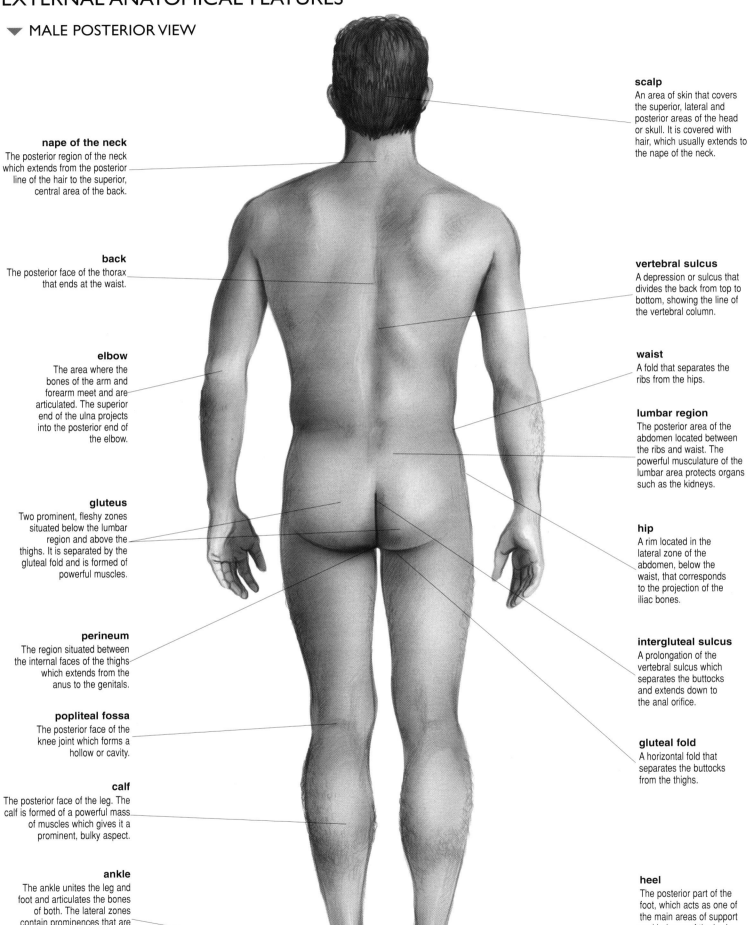

scalp
An area of skin that covers the superior, lateral and posterior areas of the head or skull. It is covered with hair, which usually extends to the nape of the neck.

nape of the neck
The posterior region of the neck which extends from the posterior line of the hair to the superior, central area of the back.

back
The posterior face of the thorax that ends at the waist.

elbow
The area where the bones of the arm and forearm meet and are articulated. The superior end of the ulna projects into the posterior end of the elbow.

gluteus
Two prominent, fleshy zones situated below the lumbar region and above the thighs. It is separated by the gluteal fold and is formed of powerful muscles.

perineum
The region situated between the internal faces of the thighs which extends from the anus to the genitals.

popliteal fossa
The posterior face of the knee joint which forms a hollow or cavity.

calf
The posterior face of the leg. The calf is formed of a powerful mass of muscles which gives it a prominent, bulky aspect.

ankle
The ankle unites the leg and foot and articulates the bones of both. The lateral zones contain prominences that are the distal portions of the tibia and fibula and are known as the malleoli.

vertebral sulcus
A depression or sulcus that divides the back from top to bottom, showing the line of the vertebral column.

waist
A fold that separates the ribs from the hips.

lumbar region
The posterior area of the abdomen located between the ribs and waist. The powerful musculature of the lumbar area protects organs such as the kidneys.

hip
A rim located in the lateral zone of the abdomen, below the waist, that corresponds to the projection of the iliac bones.

intergluteal sulcus
A prolongation of the vertebral sulcus which separates the buttocks and extends down to the anal orifice.

gluteal fold
A horizontal fold that separates the buttocks from the thighs.

heel
The posterior part of the foot, which acts as one of the main areas of support and balance of the body. The posterior prominence of the heel is the termination of the calcaneous bone.

HEAD

▼ FEMALE FRONTAL VIEW

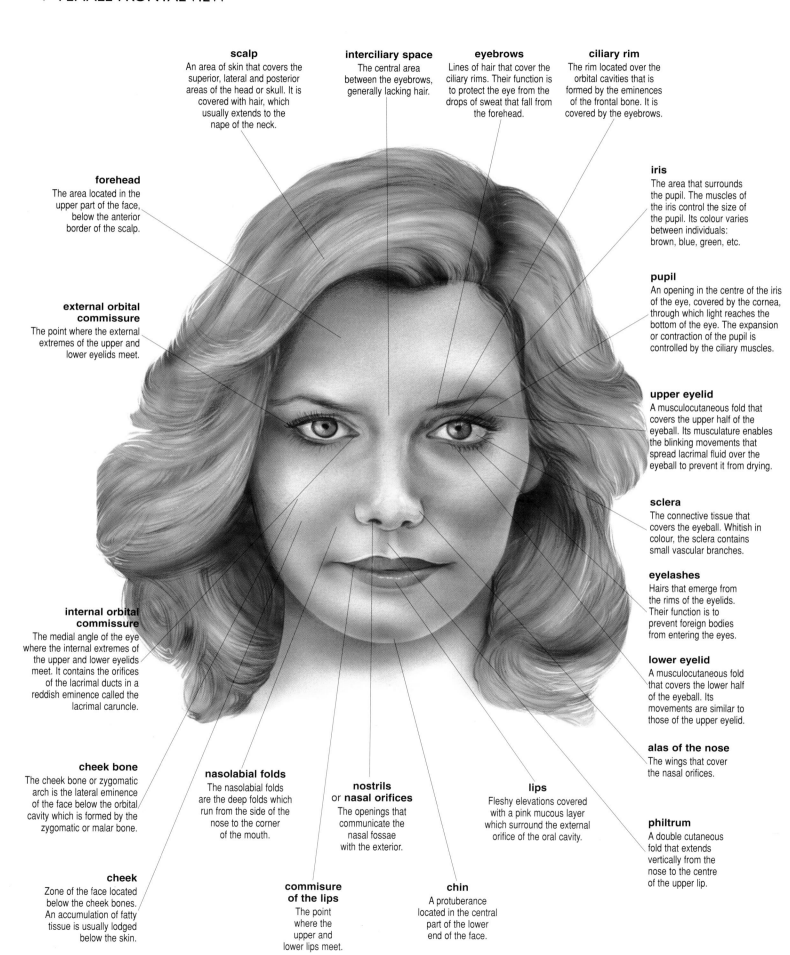

scalp
An area of skin that covers the superior, lateral and posterior areas of the head or skull. It is covered with hair, which usually extends to the nape of the neck.

interciliary space
The central area between the eyebrows, generally lacking hair.

eyebrows
Lines of hair that cover the ciliary rims. Their function is to protect the eye from the drops of sweat that fall from the forehead.

ciliary rim
The rim located over the orbital cavities that is formed by the eminences of the frontal bone. It is covered by the eyebrows.

forehead
The area located in the upper part of the face, below the anterior border of the scalp.

external orbital commissure
The point where the external extremes of the upper and lower eyelids meet.

iris
The area that surrounds the pupil. The muscles of the iris control the size of the pupil. Its colour varies between individuals: brown, blue, green, etc.

pupil
An opening in the centre of the iris of the eye, covered by the cornea, through which light reaches the bottom of the eye. The expansion or contraction of the pupil is controlled by the ciliary muscles.

upper eyelid
A musculocutaneous fold that covers the upper half of the eyeball. Its musculature enables the blinking movements that spread lacrimal fluid over the eyeball to prevent it from drying.

sclera
The connective tissue that covers the eyeball. Whitish in colour, the sclera contains small vascular branches.

eyelashes
Hairs that emerge from the rims of the eyelids. Their function is to prevent foreign bodies from entering the eyes.

internal orbital commissure
The medial angle of the eye where the internal extremes of the upper and lower eyelids meet. It contains the orifices of the lacrimal ducts in a reddish eminence called the lacrimal caruncle.

lower eyelid
A musculocutaneous fold that covers the lower half of the eyeball. Its movements are similar to those of the upper eyelid.

alas of the nose
The wings that cover the nasal orifices.

cheek bone
The cheek bone or zygomatic arch is the lateral eminence of the face below the orbital cavity which is formed by the zygomatic or malar bone.

nasolabial folds
The nasolabial folds are the deep folds which run from the side of the nose to the corner of the mouth.

nostrils or nasal orifices
The openings that communicate the nasal fossae with the exterior.

lips
Fleshy elevations covered with a pink mucous layer which surround the external orifice of the oral cavity.

philtrum
A double cutaneous fold that extends vertically from the nose to the centre of the upper lip.

cheek
Zone of the face located below the cheek bones. An accumulation of fatty tissue is usually lodged below the skin.

commisure of the lips
The point where the upper and lower lips meet.

chin
A protuberance located in the central part of the lower end of the face.

12

HEAD

▼ MALE LATERAL VIEW

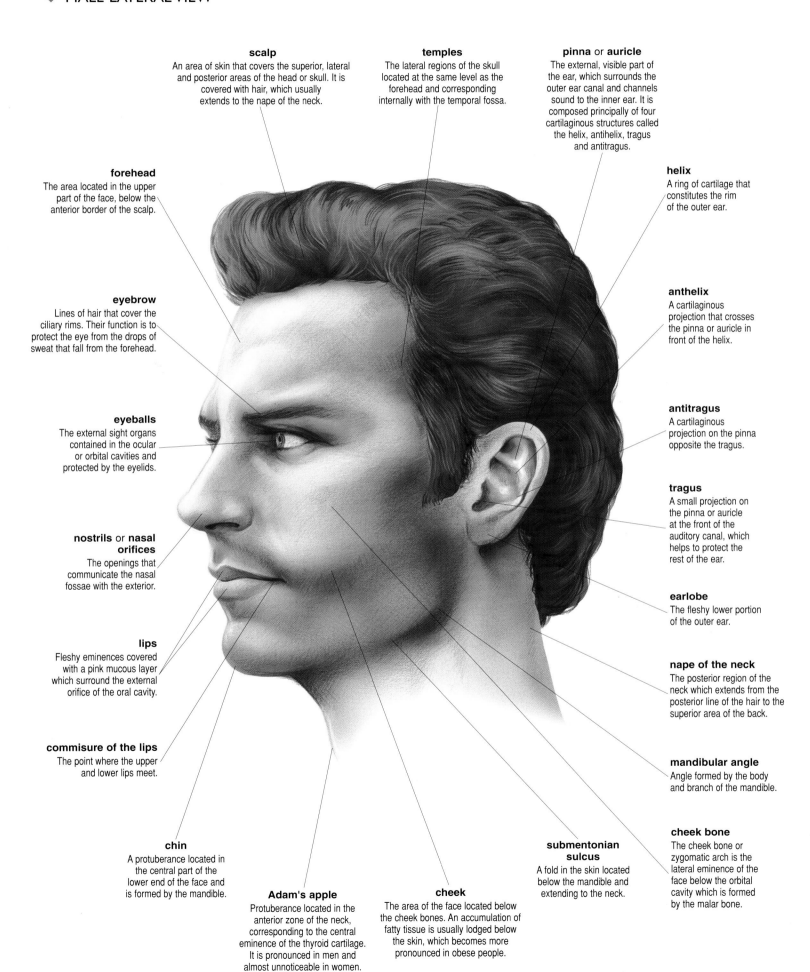

scalp
An area of skin that covers the superior, lateral and posterior areas of the head or skull. It is covered with hair, which usually extends to the nape of the neck.

temples
The lateral regions of the skull located at the same level as the forehead and corresponding internally with the temporal fossa.

pinna or **auricle**
The external, visible part of the ear, which surrounds the outer ear canal and channels sound to the inner ear. It is composed principally of four cartilaginous structures called the helix, antihelix, tragus and antitragus.

helix
A ring of cartilage that constitutes the rim of the outer ear.

forehead
The area located in the upper part of the face, below the anterior border of the scalp.

eyebrow
Lines of hair that cover the ciliary rims. Their function is to protect the eye from the drops of sweat that fall from the forehead.

anthelix
A cartilaginous projection that crosses the pinna or auricle in front of the helix.

eyeballs
The external sight organs contained in the ocular or orbital cavities and protected by the eyelids.

antitragus
A cartilaginous projection on the pinna opposite the tragus.

tragus
A small projection on the pinna or auricle at the front of the auditory canal, which helps to protect the rest of the ear.

nostrils or **nasal orifices**
The openings that communicate the nasal fossae with the exterior.

earlobe
The fleshy lower portion of the outer ear.

lips
Fleshy eminences covered with a pink mucous layer which surround the external orifice of the oral cavity.

nape of the neck
The posterior region of the neck which extends from the posterior line of the hair to the superior area of the back.

commisure of the lips
The point where the upper and lower lips meet.

mandibular angle
Angle formed by the body and branch of the mandible.

cheek bone
The cheek bone or zygomatic arch is the lateral eminence of the face below the orbital cavity which is formed by the malar bone.

chin
A protuberance located in the central part of the lower end of the face and is formed by the mandible.

submentonian sulcus
A fold in the skin located below the mandible and extending to the neck.

Adam's apple
Protuberance located in the anterior zone of the neck, corresponding to the central eminence of the thyroid cartilage. It is pronounced in men and almost unnoticeable in women.

cheek
The area of the face located below the cheek bones. An accumulation of fatty tissue is usually lodged below the skin, which becomes more pronounced in obese people.

13

THE STRUCTURE OF CELLS

nucleus
A spherical corpuscle located in the centre of the cytoplasm. It contains all the genetic material of the cell including the inherited codes that play an important role in reproduction, growth and cellular metabolism.

granular endoplasmic reticulum
A complex structure formed by multiple tubular membranes that cross all the cytoplasm; corpuscles called ribosomes adhere to its surface. It is thought to be a continuation of the nuclear membrane.

microvilli or microcilia
Prolongations emitted by the cellular membrane which enlarge the surface area of the cell, thus increasing the area of absorption, secretion, etc.

pinocytic vesicle or phagosome
A vacuole or globule formed from the cellular membrane, that, through a process known as pinocytosis, traps molecules contained in the fluid that surrounds the cell in its interior.

cellular membrane
The external layer that covers all the surface of the cell; it is elastic and permeable, allowing the products needed for the functioning of the cell to enter and waste products to be expelled. It consists of two layers of phospholipids, which are interlinked with proteins and carbohydrates.

cytoplasm or protoplasm
A fluid contained within the cellular membrane, composed of water, proteins, fats and carbohydrates and different structures or organelles, each with a specific function. The liquid part of the cytoplasm is called the cytosol.

nuclear membrane
A double layer that covers the nucleus and separates it from the cytoplasm. Its porous structure allows constant communication between both.

mitochondrion
A tubular organelle composed of two membranes. The internal membrane is folded into cristae or crests. Mitochondria play an important role in cellular respiration and the production of energy.

nucleoplasm
A fluid contained in the nuclear membrane in which the internal nuclear structures float.

ribosome
A small corpuscle that adheres to the membranes of the granular endoplasmic reticulum. In its interior, the proteins of the organism are manufactured through the combination of different amino acids.

14

smooth endoplasmic reticulum
Like the granulated endoplasmic reticulum, it is formed by membranes arranged in tubular forms in the interior of the cytoplasm, but, unlike the granular reticulum, it does not have ribosomes adhering to its membrane. Its function is the synthesis of proteins, glycoproteins and lipids.

microfilaments
The cytoplasm is furrowed by a series of microfilaments that form part of the cytoskeleton, which maintains the cell shape and aids movement.

peroxisome
A corpuscle similar to the lysosome that contains enzymes, although unlike the lysosome, the peroxisome is involved in cellular metabolism through the oxidation processes.

centrioles
Two hollow, cylindrical structures, located near the nucleus, whose walls are formed by tubular systems. Their function is cellular reproduction.

Golgi apparatus
Cavities formed of cisternae and vesicles, which are surrounded by fine membranes that unite them. Their basic function is the transport of proteins from one part of the cytoplasm to another and to the exterior of the cell.

chromosomes
Thin filaments composed of long chromatin threads. They contain the genes, which are genetic chains that store the specific inherited characteristics or traits of each individual (colour of the eyes or the hair, glandular functions, etc).

nucleolus
A spherical, intranuclear structure that plays an important role in cellular reproduction through the synthesis of nucleic acids.

flagellum
A propulsive structure used by many cells to enable them to move, by vibration or wriggling. The spermatozoa, male sexual cells, have one long tail or flagellum that equips them with great mobility.

lysosome
A vesicle containing many digestive enzymes that capture the nutritious substances contained in the phagosomes and digest them, manufacturing a part that can be used by the cell and waste products that are eliminated.

CHROMOSOMES. DNA

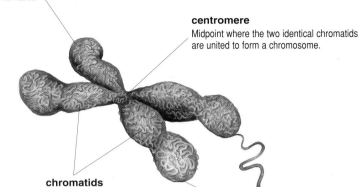

short arm
Shorter half of the two into which the centromere divides the chromatids.

centromere
Midpoint where the two identical chromatids are united to form a chromosome.

chromosomes
Structures in the cellular nucleus, visible only during the reproductive phase, when they are formed from chromatin filaments. Each chromosome is formed by two identical halves called chromatids, and thus their DNA is duplicated. Each species has a specific number of chromosomes; humans have 46, arranged in 23 pairs. Of these, 22 pairs are identical in men and women (autosomes), and there is one pair, called X (female) or Y (male) chromosomes, which define the sex (gonosomes or sexual chromosomes).

chromatids
One of the tiny (700nm) identical halves that form a chromosome. They are constituted of filaments of chromatin folded and rolled in on themselves. Each chromatid has the same DNA composition as its pair, since they will separate and contribute the same genetic load to two future cells.

long arm
Longer half of the two into which the centromere divides the chromatids.

nucleotide
One of the components of the DNA chains, nucleotides are the fragments where the phosphoric acid and deoxyribose are united with guanine, adenine, thymine or cytosine. Thus, in each DNA chain there are four different nucleotides that are repeated in a specific sequence.

nucleosomes
The double DNA helix, if unfolded, would have a length of up to 5cm (2in). In order to make it fit in a very small space, such as the nucleus, it must fold in on itself to a remarkable degree; this is accomplished by proteins called histones that, united with the DNA chains, form the nucleosomes. The DNA chains are wrapped around the histones in two turns, shortening the length of the chain considerably.

DIAGRAM OF THE DNA CHAIN

15

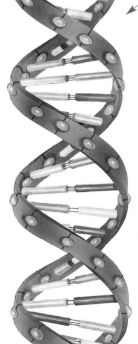

DNA
(DEOXYRIBONUCLEIC ACID)

The chromatin filaments are formed by two structures in the form of a helix, which are constituted of a skeleton composed of phosphoric acid, and a sugar, deoxyribose, to which four nitrogenated substances adhere in a specific sequence: adenine (A), guanine (G), thymine (T) and cytosine (C). In turn, the two chains are united by hydrogen bonds. It is the different combinations of these four elements (A, G, T and C) that manufacture a code that, correctly interpreted, reveals the genetic message of the cell.

THE **23** CHROMOSOMES
OF THE HUMAN KARYOTYPE

karyotype
The set of chromosomes of the human cell when they adopt a differentiated form, which can be observed in the central phases of mitosis. The dark bands correspond to groups of well-identified genes that are distributed along the long and short arms of each chromatid. Each chromosome of this map has a specific form and length, which allows its identification.

1   2   3   4   5   6

7   8   9   10   11   12

13   14   15   16   17   18

19   20   21   22   X   Y

CELLULAR REPRODUCTION

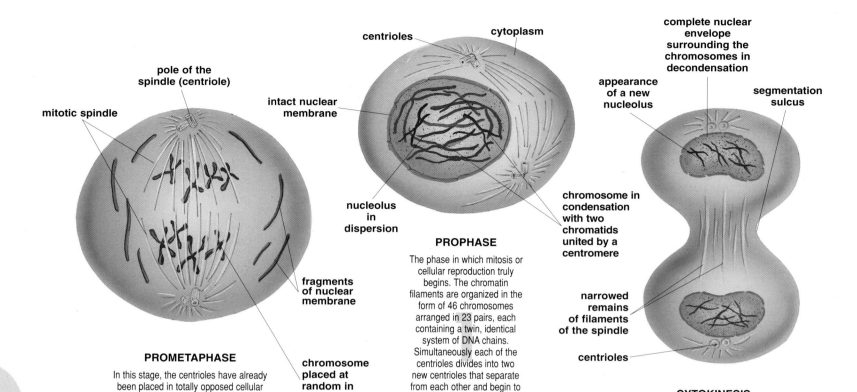

mitotic spindle

pole of the spindle (centriole)

centrioles

cytoplasm

intact nuclear membrane

complete nuclear envelope surrounding the chromosomes in decondensation

appearance of a new nucleolus

segmentation sulcus

nucleolus in dispersion

chromosome in condensation with two chromatids united by a centromere

fragments of nuclear membrane

chromosome placed at random in active movement

narrowed remains of filaments of the spindle

centrioles

PROPHASE

The phase in which mitosis or cellular reproduction truly begins. The chromatin filaments are organized in the form of 46 chromosomes arranged in 23 pairs, each containing a twin, identical system of DNA chains. Simultaneously each of the centrioles divides into two new centrioles that separate from each other and begin to migrate to opposite cellular poles.

PROMETAPHASE

In this stage, the centrioles have already been placed in totally opposed cellular poles, although they remain united by fibres composed of the tubules of the cytoskeleton that make up the mitotic spindle. Simultaneously, the nuclear membrane dissolves, the nucleolus disappears and the chromosomes are fixed to the fibres of the mitotic spindle by special structures of the centromere called kinetochores.

CYTOKINESIS

In the cellular cytoplasm, the mitotic spindles disappear and the cellular membrane begins to experience a progressive narrowing in its equatorial plane which is named the segmentation sulcus and which ends in the splitting of the mother cell into two identical cells. Inside the new nuclear membrane, the nucleoli appear. When the reproduction is finished, the cell will return to the interphase or non-reproductive period.

PHASES OF MITOSIS

Mitosis is the form of cellular reproduction which enables the cell to divide after duplicating its genetic load, so that each daughter cell receives a complete set of chromosomes.

stationary chromosomes aligned in the metaphasic plate equidistant from the poles

fragment of nuclear envelope

chromosomes (chromatids) in the decondensation phase

kinetochores

separated chromatid attracted towards the pole

nuclear envelope in the phase of formation around each chromosome

pole of the spindle

METAPHASE

Once the centrioles have been placed in totally opposed planes of the cell and the chromosomes have been united to the fibres of the mitotic spindle by the kinetochores, each of the two centrioles begins to exert an attraction of equal intensity on the chromosomes and, consequently, these migrate to the equatorial plane of the cell, constituting an equatorial or metaphasic plate.

ANAPHASE

During the anaphase, the attraction of the centrioles on the chromosomes becomes more intense, so that each pair of chromosomes is divided by its centromere into two halves and each of these initiates a migration towards an opposed cellular pole, while the cell becomes elongated, increasing the distance between the poles.

TELOPHASE

In this phase, the chromosomes are organized around each centriole, while around them a membranous structure, the future nuclear membrane, begins to form. At the end of the telophase, the chromosomes begin to become disorganized and adopt the diffuse chromatin form again.

16

BODY TISSUES

TISSUES

The cells of the human body are grouped together to form more complicated structures called tissues. These are the elements from which the different systems that form the human body are constructed. There are seven types of body tissue.

PAVEMENT EPITHELIA

simple epithelium

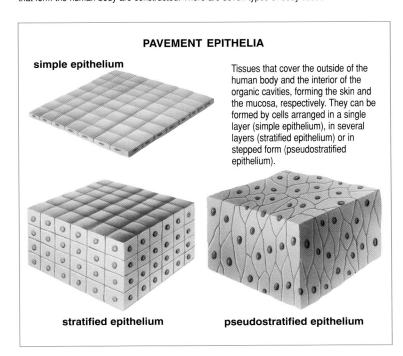

Tissues that cover the outside of the human body and the interior of the organic cavities, forming the skin and the mucosa, respectively. They can be formed by cells arranged in a single layer (simple epithelium), in several layers (stratified epithelium) or in stepped form (pseudostratified epithelium).

stratified epithelium   **pseudostratified epithelium**

GLANDULAR EPITHELIA

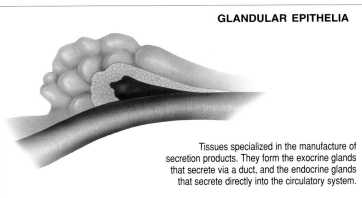

Tissues specialized in the manufacture of secretion products. They form the exocrine glands that secrete via a duct, and the endocrine glands that secrete directly into the circulatory system.

NERVOUS TISSUE

A specialized tissue that permits the transmission of the neuroelectrical impulses which constitute the basis of all the governing functions of the nervous system, allowing the brain to transmit its orders. The brain, cerebellum, spinal marrow and all the nerves of the organism are composed of nervous tissue.

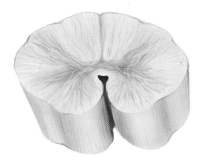

CONNECTIVE TISSUE

There are various types of connective tissue, also known as conjunctive tissue.

LOOSE TISSUE

The matrix on which most organs are constructed (liver, alimentary canal, lungs, etc.). It forms part of the internal membranes and fills the space that exists among them; it is formed by cells called fibroblasts, a fundamental substance composed of water, mineral sugars and salts, and fibres of collagen, reticulin and elastin.

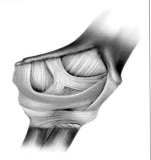

DENSE TISSUE

Dense tissue acts as a support and forms the structure of bones, tendons, ligaments, blood vessels, etc. Its structure is similar to that of loose connective tissue, but the proportion of constituent fibres varies.

ADIPOSE TISSUE

Adipose tissue is the body's fat store and is an important reserve of energy and a protective cushion for the internal organs. It is formed by cells rich in fatty material, the adipocytes.

BLOOD

This tissue is the body's method of transporting the substances necessary for the sustenance of its cells to all parts of the body and of ridding the organs of metabolic waste products. It is composed of a liquid (plasma) and solids (blood cells).

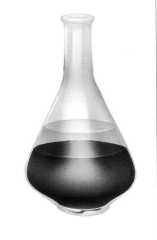

LYMPHOID TISSUE

The tissue specialized in the production of cells that form the body's defence mechanisms (lymphocytes, plasmacytes, etc.), which combat foreign bodies such as bacteria, viruses, etc. It is found in the lymphoid organs, which are the lymph nodes, the bone marrow and the tonsils.

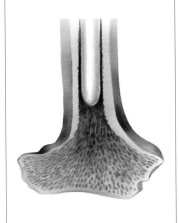

17

MUSCULAR TISSUE

The tissue that forms muscles which, through their contraction, are able to develop mechanical functions. Smooth muscular tissue is contracted involuntarily and is found in internal organs such as the intestine, uterus and arteries. Striated muscular tissue contracts voluntarily, and is found in the muscles of the extremities, neck, thorax, abdomen, etc.

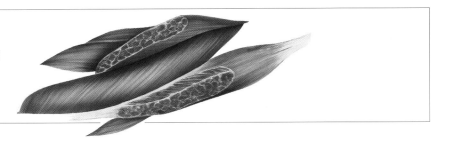

MICROSCOPIC STRUCTURE OF THE SKIN

epidermis
The outermost of the three layers of the skin. It consists of five strata in which the epidermic cells, the keratinocytes, gradually evolve and harden progressively by the process known as keratinization.

dermis
The layer of the skin located below the epidermis and composed of loose connective tissue and fibrous tissue. It contains many nerve terminations and blood vessels. In this layer, the sudoriferous glands, the sebaceous glands and the roots of the hair and different types of cell such as fibroblasts, histiocytes and mastocytes are located.

hypodermis
The deepest layer of the skin, located below the dermis. It is formed of loose connective tissue and contains abundant adipose tissue, which acts as a cushion for the organs below (muscles, bones, viscera, etc.), from which it is separated by the subcutaneous cellular tissue, the deepest portion of the hypodermis.

basal layer
Also known as the germinative layer, it is located in the deepest part, and continuously produces new keratinocytes.

spinous layer
Located above the basal layer and composed of continuously multiplying keratinocytes.

granular layer
Formed of epidermic cells that initiate their cornification or hardening.

clear layer
The clear layer only exists in zones of very compact skin and is formed by flattened, dead keratinocytes.

horny layer
Superficial layer of the epidermis, where the keratinized epidermic cells are shed and replaced by others. The soles of the feet and the palms of the hands have a thicker layer.

pores
Small openings that sometimes coincide with the superior end of the excretory channel of a sudoriferous gland or with the birth of a hair.

keratinocytes
The cells that form the epidermis. They originate in the basal layer and evolve continuously to terminate as dead cells which are shed by the corneous layer.

dermal papillae
Superior part of the dermis, formed by small nipple-like protrusions that extend into the epidermis.

blood capillaries

18

epidermis

dermis

hypodermis

Paccini's corpuscle
Nervous terminations located in the deepest part of the dermis that detect the deepest tactile sensations.

Meissner's corpuscle
Nervous terminations of the dermis that detect superficial tactile sensations. They are very abundant in the fingertips.

Ruffini's corpuscle
Nervous terminations of the dermis specialized in detecting heat.

Krause's corpuscle
Nervous terminations of the dermis that detect cold sensations.

sudoriferous gland
Glandular structures in the form of a twisted tubule, specialized in the secretion of sweat. They are located in the sinus of the dermis and expel their secretions through a duct that opens to the epidermis through the pores.

erector muscle of the hair
A thin muscle that unites the base of the hair follicle with the epidermis. Its function is to facilitate the erection of the hair in situations of cold, stress, etc.

Langerhan's cells
Cells located in the spinous layer between the keratinocytes. Morphologically, they resemble melanocytes.

melanocytes
Cells located between the keratinocytes of the basal layer. Their function is to synthesize melanin, the substance responsible for the colour of the skin and the hair, which is a powerful protective filter of solar rays.

hair follicle
A saccular structure that contains the hair and the sebaceous glands.

ACCESSORY ORGANS OF THE SKIN. HAIR FOLLICLE

CROSS-SECTION OF A FOLLICLE

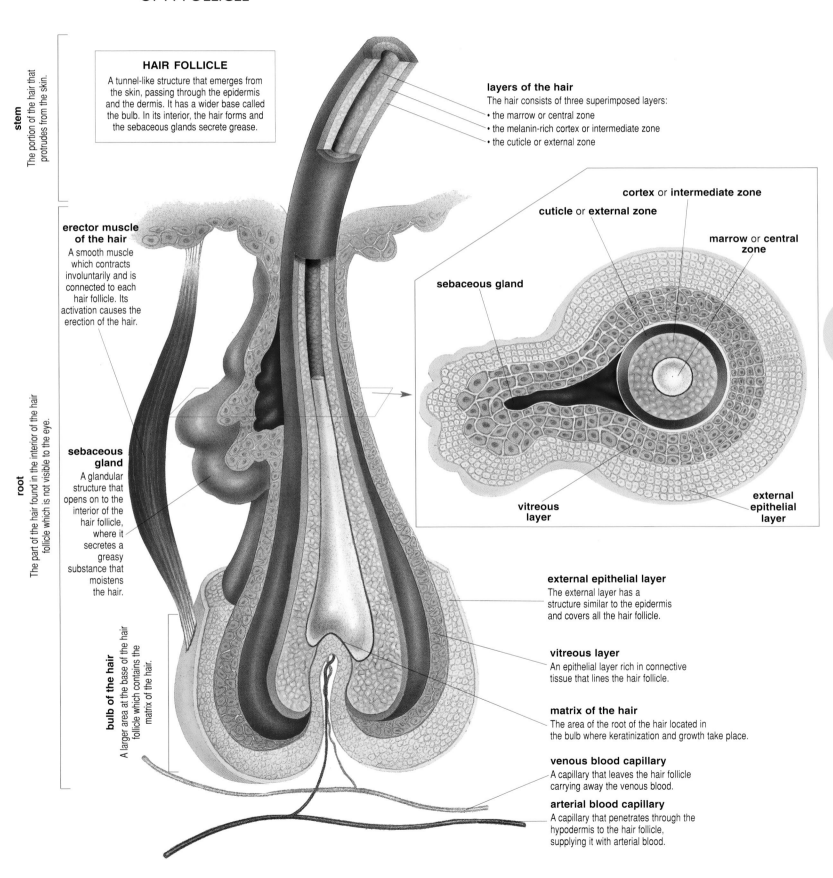

stem
The portion of the hair that protrudes from the skin.

root
The part of the hair found in the interior of the hair follicle which is not visible to the eye.

HAIR FOLLICLE
A tunnel-like structure that emerges from the skin, passing through the epidermis and the dermis. It has a wider base called the bulb. In its interior, the hair forms and the sebaceous glands secrete grease.

layers of the hair
The hair consists of three superimposed layers:
• the marrow or central zone
• the melanin-rich cortex or intermediate zone
• the cuticle or external zone

erector muscle of the hair
A smooth muscle which contracts involuntarily and is connected to each hair follicle. Its activation causes the erection of the hair.

sebaceous gland
A glandular structure that opens on to the interior of the hair follicle, where it secretes a greasy substance that moistens the hair.

bulb of the hair
A larger area at the base of the hair follicle which contains the matrix of the hair.

cortex or **intermediate zone**

cuticle or **external zone**

marrow or **central zone**

sebaceous gland

external epithelial layer

vitreous layer

external epithelial layer
The external layer has a structure similar to the epidermis and covers all the hair follicle.

vitreous layer
An epithelial layer rich in connective tissue that lines the hair follicle.

matrix of the hair
The area of the root of the hair located in the bulb where keratinization and growth take place.

venous blood capillary
A capillary that leaves the hair follicle carrying away the venous blood.

arterial blood capillary
A capillary that penetrates through the hypodermis to the hair follicle, supplying it with arterial blood.

19

ACCESSORY ORGANS OF THE SKIN. FINGERNAIL

**body of the nail
or ungueal limb**
The visible part of the fingernail located in the posterior face of the distal extremity of the fingers. It is hard and horny and is formed of keratinized epithelial cells.

periungual fold
A fold of skin that surrounds the lateral parts of the body of the nail. The fold can allow infections, known as panaris infections, to enter.

lunula
An area of the nail with a clearer colour and semicircular edge located at the base of the body of the nail.

cuticle
Whitish, soft, membranous lamina that surrounds the body of the nail body at its base, in the area of the lunula, and separates it from the surrounding skin.

ungual root
The newest part of the nail which is contained in the matrix.

matrix of the nail
An area located under the skin of the ends of the fingers which contains the epithelial cells which, through the process of keratinization, form the nail.

nail bed
The portion of skin on which the nail rests and which serves as a base.

free edge
The distal end of the body of the nail that, due to its growth, is continually approaching the end of the finger.

perionychium
An area of skin that separates the nail bed of the epidermis from the fingertip.

**striae
of the nails**
Fine whitish lines that sometimes appear on the body of the nail. They are due to stratification defects in the keratinized cells that form the nail.

distal phalange
The last of the phalangeal bones that supports the structure of the nail and finger.

fingertip
The area located at the anterior distal ends of the fingers. It contains characteristic cutaneous sulci that are called dermatoglyphs and which are the origin of fingerprints.

subcutaneous fat
An accumulation of adipose tissue located under the layers of the skin, specifically in contact with the hypodermis, for which it forms the cushioning.

20

ACCESSORY ORGANS OF THE SKIN. SUDORIFEROUS GLANDS

SWEAT

The secretion produced by the sudoriferous glands. It is mainly composed of water which contains large amounts of dissolved minerals. The evaporation of sweat plays an important role in regulating the temperature of the body.

epidermis

dermis

hypodermis

external layer of the sudoriferous gland
A layer of myoepithelial cells that covers all the sudoriferous gland.

internal layer of the sudoriferous gland
A layer of epithelial cells that is bistratified in the excretory tubule and monostratified in the secretory portion. It forms the internal lining of the sudoriferous gland.

blood capillaries
Small blood capillaries that carry blood to the base of the secretory portion of the gland.

sympathetic nervous termination
The sudoriferous glands are controlled by the vegetative nervous system, and thus receive a nervous termination from the sympathetic system.

pore
The external orifice of the sudoriferous gland that connects with the exterior. It secretes sweat and is usually located close to a hair follicle.

excretory duct
A tubular system which, starting in the secretory portion, rises in a spiral trajectory and terminates in the epidermis.

secretory portion
The deepest part of the dermis formed by coiled ducts lined with cells specialized in producing sweat.

21

COMPOSITION OF SWEAT

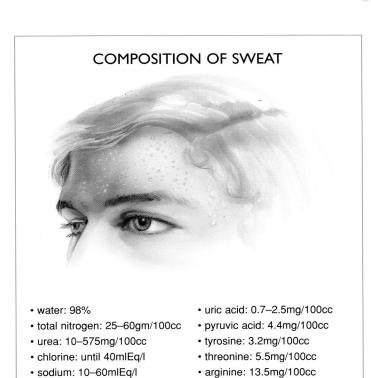

- water: 98%
- total nitrogen: 25–60gm/100cc
- urea: 10–575mg/100cc
- chlorine: until 40mlEq/l
- sodium: 10–60mlEq/l
- potassium: 3–10mlEq/l
- lactic acid: 45–450mg/100cc

- uric acid: 0.7–2.5mg/100cc
- pyruvic acid: 4.4mg/100cc
- tyrosine: 3.2mg/100cc
- threonine: 5.5mg/100cc
- arginine: 13.5mg/100cc
- histidine: 8mg/100cc

DISTRIBUTION OF THE SUDORIFEROUS GLANDS

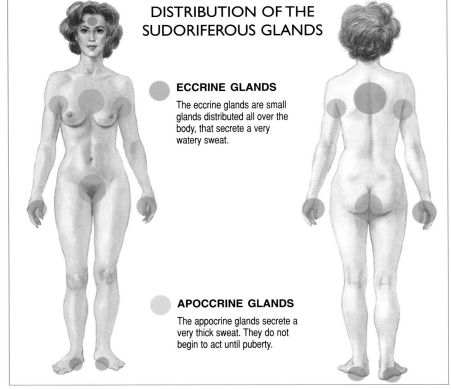

ECCRINE GLANDS

The eccrine glands are small glands distributed all over the body, that secrete a very watery sweat.

APOCCRINE GLANDS

The appocrine glands secrete a very thick sweat. They do not begin to act until puberty.

MUSCULAR SYSTEM

▼ GENERAL ANTERIOR VIEW

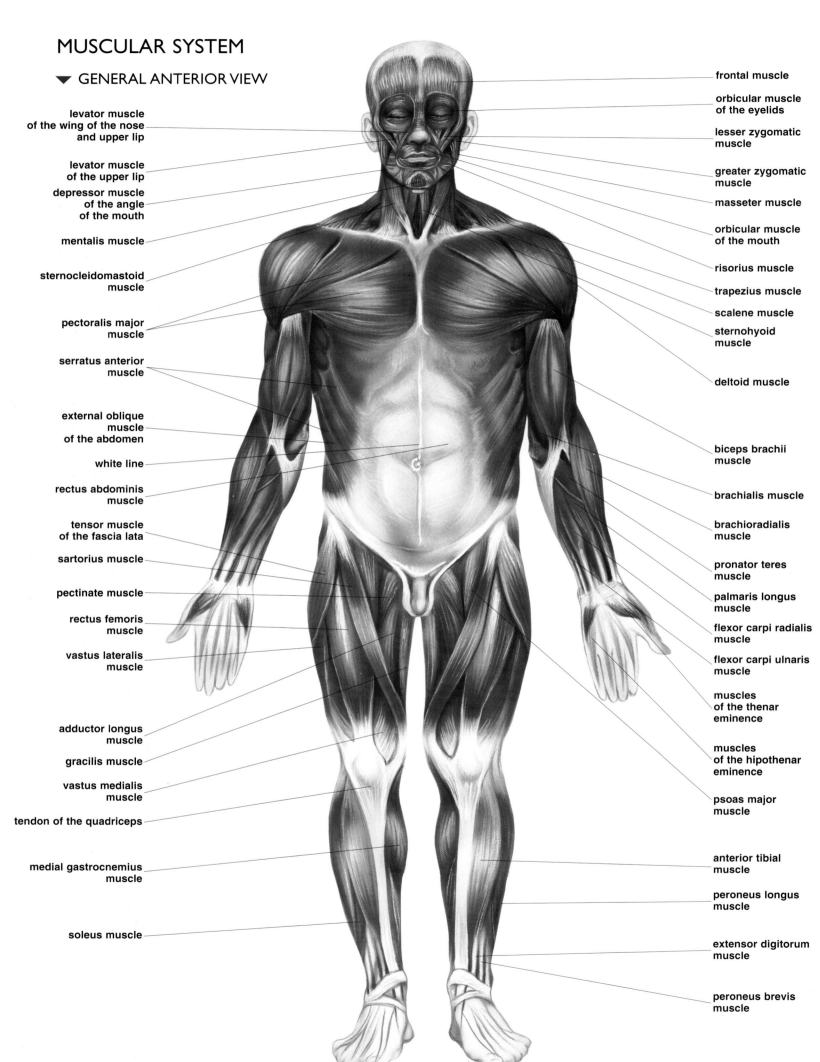

levator muscle
of the wing of the nose
and upper lip

levator muscle
of the upper lip

depressor muscle
of the angle
of the mouth

mentalis muscle

sternocleidomastoid
muscle

pectoralis major
muscle

serratus anterior
muscle

external oblique
muscle
of the abdomen

white line

rectus abdominis
muscle

tensor muscle
of the fascia lata

sartorius muscle

pectinate muscle

rectus femoris
muscle

vastus lateralis
muscle

adductor longus
muscle

gracilis muscle

vastus medialis
muscle

tendon of the quadriceps

medial gastrocnemius
muscle

soleus muscle

frontal muscle

orbicular muscle
of the eyelids

lesser zygomatic
muscle

greater zygomatic
muscle

masseter muscle

orbicular muscle
of the mouth

risorius muscle

trapezius muscle

scalene muscle

sternohyoid
muscle

deltoid muscle

biceps brachii
muscle

brachialis muscle

brachioradialis
muscle

pronator teres
muscle

palmaris longus
muscle

flexor carpi radialis
muscle

flexor carpi ulnaris
muscle

muscles
of the thenar
eminence

muscles
of the hipothenar
eminence

psoas major
muscle

anterior tibial
muscle

peroneus longus
muscle

extensor digitorum
muscle

peroneus brevis
muscle

MUSCULAR SYSTEM

▼ POSTERIOR GENERAL VIEW

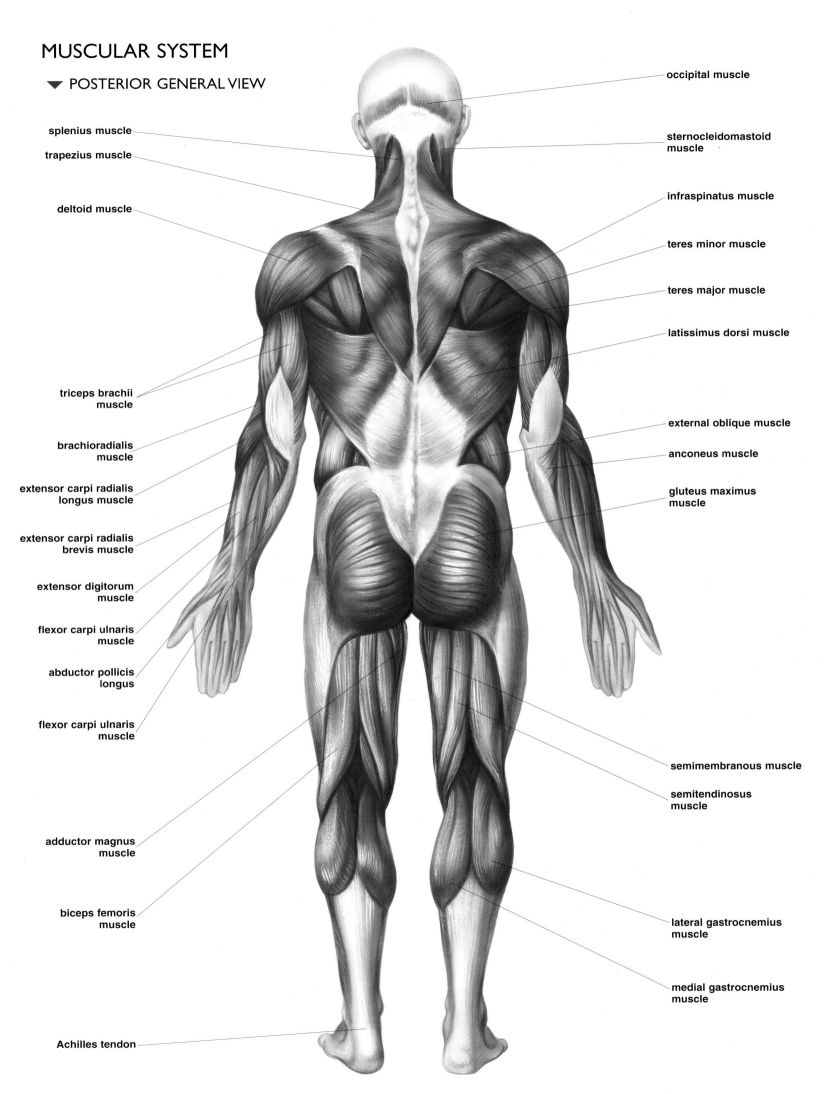

splenius muscle

trapezius muscle

deltoid muscle

triceps brachii muscle

brachioradialis muscle

extensor carpi radialis longus muscle

extensor carpi radialis brevis muscle

extensor digitorum muscle

flexor carpi ulnaris muscle

abductor pollicis longus

flexor carpi ulnaris muscle

adductor magnus muscle

biceps femoris muscle

Achilles tendon

occipital muscle

sternocleidomastoid muscle

infraspinatus muscle

teres minor muscle

teres major muscle

latissimus dorsi muscle

external oblique muscle

anconeus muscle

gluteus maximus muscle

semimembranous muscle

semitendinosus muscle

lateral gastrocnemius muscle

medial gastrocnemius muscle

23

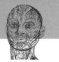
EXTERNAL AND INTERNAL STRUCTURE OF A STRIATED MUSCLE

insertion points
The points at which the tendons are fixed to the skeleton, allowing muscular contractions to be transmitted to bones, cartilages or joints to enable movement.

tendons
Found at the extremes of almost all striated muscles, tendons serve as fixation elements between the muscles and skeleton. They are formed of pearly coloured fibrous connective tissue.

containment aponeurosis
Membranous sheaths that surround striated muscles and separate the different muscular groups. They are formed of fibrous connective tissue similar to that of the tendons.

muscular belly
The most voluminous part of the muscle, almost always located in the centre of the muscle.

blood vessels
The muscles are supplied by arteries that carry oxygenated blood via capillaries to veins that carry the deoxygenated blood away to the venous network.

somatic nerve
The brain sends nervous impulses that stimulate voluntary movements to the muscle through the somatic nerve.

STRIATED MUSCLE

The striated or skeletal muscles are those that move voluntarily, following a conscious order from the brain. They are transmitted through the somatic nerves and are attached to the different parts of the skeleton, allowing movement.

---

myofibrils
Small cylindrical filaments measuring 1–2 micrometers in diameter. Each muscular fibre contains thousands.

endomysium
Very fine layer of reticular fibres that originate in the perimysium and surround each of the muscular fibres that make up the muscle.

epimysium
Membranous connective tissue that surrounds the muscle and whose prolongations form part of the tendons.

sarcolemma
The plasma membrane that surrounds each cell or muscular fibre.

blood capillaries
Small capillaries that provide the blood flow to the muscular fibres through the perimysium.

muscular fibres
Cells or structural units arranged longitudinally within the muscle. Their diameter ranges between 18–80 microns. They contain a fluid medium called sarcoplasm and myofibrils.

perimysium
Membranous walls that originate in the epimysium and surround a fascicle or packet of muscular fibres.

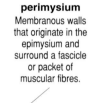

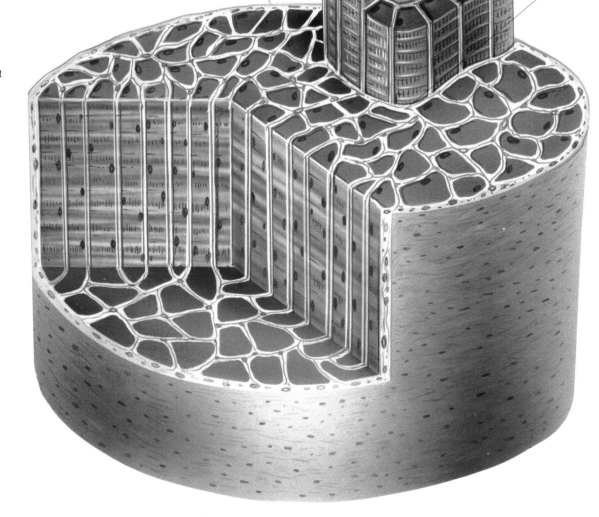

EXTERNAL AND INTERNAL STRUCTURE OF A SMOOTH MUSCLE

SMOOTH MUSCLES

Also called visceral muscles, smooth muscles move involuntarily, following automatic impulses generated in the central nervous system and transmitted through the vegetative or autonomous nervous system, without conscious thought. The smooth muscles are found in the walls of the visceral organs such as the blood vessels, intestine, bronchi, etc. and in the skin and eyes. They allow these organs to function equally during sleep or waking.

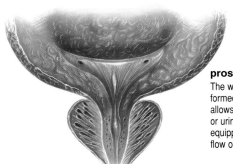

prostate and vesicle musculature
The walls of the bladder and prostate are formed of a muscular layer whose contraction allows the mechanisms triggering ejaculation or urination to occur. The bladder is also equipped with striated muscles that allow the flow of urine to be controlled voluntarily.

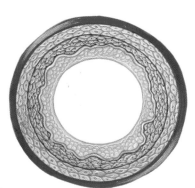

musculature of the arterial walls
The musculature of the walls of the arteries allows them to change diameter in response to the blood flow and changes in blood pressure.

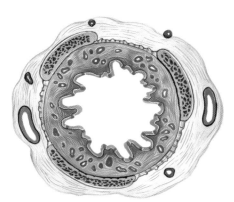

musculature of the bronchial walls
The walls of the bronchi are equipped with a muscular layer that, through relaxation or contraction, allows the bronchi to widen or narrow, enabling greater or smaller air intake to the pulmonary alveoli.

25

smooth muscular fibre
The smooth muscle is formed by bundles of fusiform cells of 80–200um in length, generally arranged in layers, especially in the walls of hollow organs (intestine, blood vessels, bronchi, etc.). It is also found in the connective tissue that lines organs such as the prostate, or forming individualized units such as the erector muscles of the hair or the muscles of the iris.

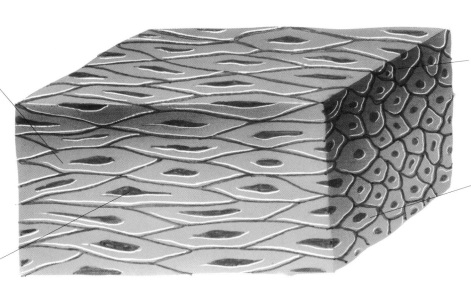

plasma membrane
Fine membrane that surrounds smooth muscle fibres. It contains a network of reticular fibres that join the muscle fibres.

sarcoplasm
Cytoplasm of smooth muscular fibre cells, which contain many tiny myofibrils, arranged irregularly and visible only under the electron microscope. The myofibrils are composed of actin and myosin and are responsible for muscular contraction.

nucleus
The cells of the smooth musculature have a single nucleus normally located in the centre of the cytoplasm.

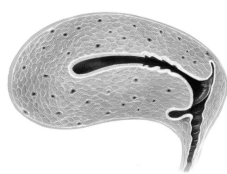

musculature of the uterine wall
The mechanisms of childbirth are possible due to the contractions of the powerful musculature of the uterine wall, which are triggered by hormonal stimuli.

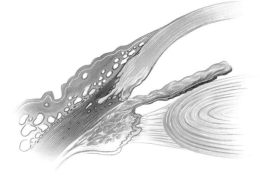

ciliary musculature of the eye
Surrounding the lens of the eye, the ciliary muscles contract or relax, allowing the shape of the lens to change and thus optimizing the vision.

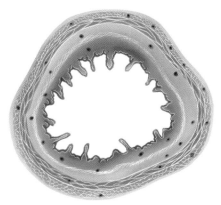

musculature of the intestinal walls
The contraction of this musculature causes the peristaltic movements that allow the nutritional bolus to advance through the different segments of the alimentary canal.

THE SKULL AND FACE. SUPERFICIAL MUSCLES

▼ FRONTAL VIEW

galea aponeurotica
A fibrous membrane that surrounds the superior area of the skull and is firmly joined to the skin that covers it, allowing it to slide over the bone. It serves as the origin of the various cutaneous muscles of the skull.

frontal muscle
A muscle that extends under the skin of the forehead, from the galea aponeurotica to the superior border of the orbit. When contracted, it tenses the galea aponeurotica, but also intervenes in facial gestures such as raising the eyebrows and making frown lines appear.

superciliary muscle
A small, thin facial muscle located below the orbicular muscle of the eyelids and the frontal, in the internal area of the superciliary arch. Its contraction allows frowning.

pyramidal muscle
A facial muscle that extends vertically along the dorsal area of the nose, from the internal ciliary area to the cartilages and bones that form the nasal skeleton. Its contraction causes the appearance of cutaneous folds between the eyebrows.

orbicular muscle of the eyelids
A circular facial muscle that surrounds the palpebral opening. It extends from the internal angle of the eye to the external angle, attached to the skin of the eyelids. It permits the opening and closing of the eyelid, allowing gestures such as winking and blinking.

levator muscle of the ala of the nose and upper lip
A facial muscle inserted in the internal area of the superior maxillary bone. From there it divides into two fascicles: one goes to the skin of the ala of the nose and the other goes to the skin of the upper lip. Its contraction elevates the ala of the nose, expands the nasal orifice and causes the upper lip to protrude upwards.

nasal muscle
Also known as the transverse muscle of the nose. A facial muscle that extends from the median line of the nasal cartilages to the skin that covers the alas of the nose. When contracted, it causes the nasal orifices to narrow and vertical facial folds to appear.

lesser zygomatic muscle
A facial muscle that extends from the zygomatic bone on one side and in the skin of the upper lip, which it elevates and turns outwards when contracted, on the other.

levator muscle of the angle of the mouth
Also known as the *canine muscle*, it extends from the zygomatic bone to the skin of the commissure of the lips, which it elevates when contracted.

greater zygomatic muscle
A long, thin facial muscle that extends from the zygomatic bone to the skin of the commissure of the lips. When contracted, it elevates the commissure, complementing the action of the levator muscle of the angle of the mouth.

buccinator muscle
A facial muscle inserted in the skin surrounding the commissure of the lips, and which extends across the cheeks to the superior border of the mandible and the inferior border of the maxilla. Its main action is to widen the commissure of the lips transversally, but it also collaborates with other muscles in blowing, whistling or chewing.

risorius muscle
A facial muscle that, by elevating the commissure of the lips upwards and outwards, allows smiling. It is inserted in the internal part of the skin of the parotid area and from there its fibres converge towards the commissure of the lips.

depressor muscle of the angle of the mouth
Also called the *triangular muscle of the lips*, due to its shape. It is attached to the inferior border of the mandible and the superior vertex located in the skin of the commissure of the lips. Its contraction allows the commissure of the lips to move downwards, permitting expressions of disgust or sadness.

platysma
A facial muscle that extends over the lateral part of the neck. Located in a very superficial position, right under the skin, it extends from near the lower lip and the chin to the skin that covers the clavicle. When contracted, it forces the skin of the chin and the lower lip downwards, collaborating with the depressor muscle of the angle of the mouth in forming expressions of loathing or sadness.

depressor muscle of the lower lip
A muscle that is inserted in the inferior border of the bone of the chin; its fibres are fixed in the skin that covers the lower lip. This muscle allows the lower lip to turn downwards and outwards.

mentalis muscle
Small facial muscle located in the lateral part of the chin. It is inserted in the external face of the bone that forms the chin and terminates in the skin of this area, so that its contraction elevates the chin.

orbicular muscle of the mouth
An elliptical facial muscle that extends from one commissure of the lips to the other by means of two fascicles, one superior and the other inferior, that cross both lips internally, leaving the buccal opening in the middle. In the commissures, the muscle is inserted in the skin of the area and in the corresponding maxillary bones. It allows the opening and closing of the mouth and it collaborates with other muscles to produce blowing, sucking and whistling actions, among others.

levator muscle of the upper lip
A facial muscle that goes from the area of the maxilla located under the orbit to the upper lip, elevating the central part of the upper lip when contracted.

26

THE SKULL AND FACE. SUPERFICIAL MUSCLES

▼ LATERAL VIEW

temporal muscle
A wide fan-shaped muscle extending from the temporal fossa to the coronoid process of the mandible which acts to raise the mandible and close the jaws, permitting the action of chewing.

frontal muscle
A muscle that extends under the skin of the forehead, from the galea aponeurotica to the superior border of the orbit. When contracted, it tenses the galea aponeurotica, but also intervenes in facial gestures such as raising the eyebrows and making frown lines appear.

temporal fascia
A fibrous lamina that covers the temporal fossa and surrounds the temporal muscle.

galea aponeurotica
A fibrous membrane that surrounds the superior area of the skull and is firmly joined to the skin that covers it, allowing it to slide over the bone. It serves as the origin of the various cutaneous muscles of the skull.

superior auricular muscle
A flat, almost atrophic muscle, located above the auricular pavilion. It goes from the lateral border of the galea aponeurotica to the superior area of the auricular cartilages, which it moves slightly upwards when contracted. There are also anterior and posterior auricular muscles.

superciliary muscle
A small, thin facial muscle located above the orbicular muscle of the eyelids and the frontal, in the internal area of the superciliary arch. Its contraction allows frowning.

orbicular muscle of the eyelids
A circular facial muscle that surrounds the palpebral opening. It extends from the internal angle of the eye to the external angle, attached to the skin of the eyelids. It permits the opening and closing of the eyelid, allowing gestures such as winking and blinking.

occipital muscle
A flat muscle composed of two parts which originates in the galea aponeurotica, and extends posteriorly to reach the lateral areas of the occipital bone. Its contraction tenses the galea aponeurotica, which covers the skull.

27

levator muscle of the ala of the nose and upper lip
A facial muscle inserted in the internal area of the superior maxillary bone. From there it divides into two fascicles: one goes to the skin of the ala of the nose and the other goes to the skin of the upper lip. Its contraction elevates the ala of the nose, expands the nasal orifice and causes the upper lip to protrude upwards.

greater zygomatic muscle
A long, thin facial muscle that goes from the cheek of the zygomatic bone to the skin of the commissure of the lips. When contracted, it elevates the commissure, complementing the action of the levator muscle of the angle of the mouth.

orbicular muscle of the mouth
An elliptical facial muscle that extends from one commissure of the lips to the other by means of two fascicles, one superior and the other inferior, that cross both lips internally, leaving the buccal opening in the middle. In the commissures, the muscle is inserted in the skin of the area and in the corresponding maxillary bones. It allows the opening and closing of the mouth and it collaborates with other muscles to produce blowing, sucking and whistling actions, among others.

sternocleidomastoid muscle
A muscle that originates in the mastoid process of the temporal and occipital bones of the head. It descends forming two fascicles: one goes to the manubrium of the sternum and the other to the clavicle. Its action is to flex, lateralize and rotate the neck.

depressor muscle of the lower lip
A muscle that is inserted in the inferior border of the bone of the chin and its fibers are fixed in the skin that covers the lower lip. This muscle allows the lower lip to turn downwards and outwards.

lesser zygomatic muscle
A facial muscle that extends from the zygomatic bone to the skin of the upper lip, which it elevates and turns outwards when contracted, on the other.

buccinator muscle
A facial muscle inserted in the skin surrounding the commissure of the lips, and which extends across the internal face of the cheeks to the superior border of the mandible and the inferior border of the maxilla. Its main action is to widen the commissure of the lips transversally, but it also collaborates with other muscles in blowing, whistling or chewing.

risorius muscle
A facial muscle that, by elevating the commissure of the lips upwards and outwards, allows smiling. It is inserted in the internal part of the skin of the parotid area and from there its fibers converge towards the commissure of the lips.

masseter muscle
One of muscles used in chewing, the masseter muscle consists of two fascicles that go from the zygomatic arch of the face bones to the angle and the ascending branch of the mandible. Its action is to elevate the mandible, meaning it is essential for chewing.

trapezius muscle
A very wide triangular muscle that covers almost all the other muscles of the nape of the neck and a large part of the back. It is inserted in the occipital bone and the spinous processes of the cervical and dorsal vertebrae, and from there it converges on the shoulder where it is inserted in the scapula and the clavicle. Its action is to elevate the shoulder and also to incline the head sideways.

THE NAPE OF THE NECK

▼ POSTERIOR VIEW

inferior oblique muscle of the head
Also known as the *greater oblique muscle*. It extends from the spinous process of the axis to the transverse process of the atlas. Its action is to rotate the head to each side.

rectus capitis posterior minor muscle
A muscle that extends from the atlas to the occipital bone and contributes to the inclination of the head backwards and sideways.

rectus capitis posterior major muscle
A flat muscle that unites the axis with the occipital bone. Its action is to help in the inclination of the head backwards and sideways and in its rotation.

galea aponeurotica
A fibrous membrane that surrounds the superior area of the skull and is firmly joined to the skin that covers it.

occipital muscle
A flat muscle that originates in the galea aponeurotica and extends to the lateral areas of the occipital bone. Its contraction tenses the skin of the skull.

semispinalis capitis muscle
A muscle that extends from the last cervical vertebrae and first dorsal vertebrae to the occipital bone. It can incline the head backwards or rotate it.

superior oblique muscle of the head
This muscle is also known as the *lesser oblique muscle*. It originates in the atlas and inserts in the occipital bone. It inclines the head laterally.

splenius muscle
A muscle located below the trapezius muscle which has a twin superior origin. One head originates in the mastoid process of the temporal bone of the skull (splenius muscle of the head), and the other originates in the first cervical vertebrae (splenius muscle of the neck). Both descend and unite to be inserted in the last cervical vertebrae and the first dorsal vertebrae. They act to incline the head backwards or laterally, or to rotate it.

semispinalis capitis
The semispinalis capitis is a muscle that goes from the last cervical vertebrae to the mastoid process of the temporal bone. Its action is to incline the head backwards and to one side.

sternocleidomastoid muscle
A muscle that originates in the mastoid process of the temporal and occipital bones of the head. It descends forming two heads: one goes to the manubrium of the sternum and the other to the clavicle. Its action is to flex, lateralize and rotate the neck.

longissimus muscle
An elongated muscle that unites the last cervical vertebrae and the first dorsal vertebrae with the mastoid process of the temporal bone. Its action is to incline the head backwards or to one side.

trapezius muscle
A very wide triangular muscle that covers almost all the other muscles of the nape of the neck and a large part of the back. It is inserted in the occipital bone and the spinous processes of the cervical and dorsal vertebrae, and from there it converges on the shoulder where it is inserted in the scapula and the clavicle. Its action is to elevate the shoulder and to incline the head sideways.

superficial cervical fascia
A thin membrane or aponeurosis that covers all the structures of the neck, emitting individual prolongations that surround some muscles of the region.

THE NECK

▼ ANTERIOR VIEW

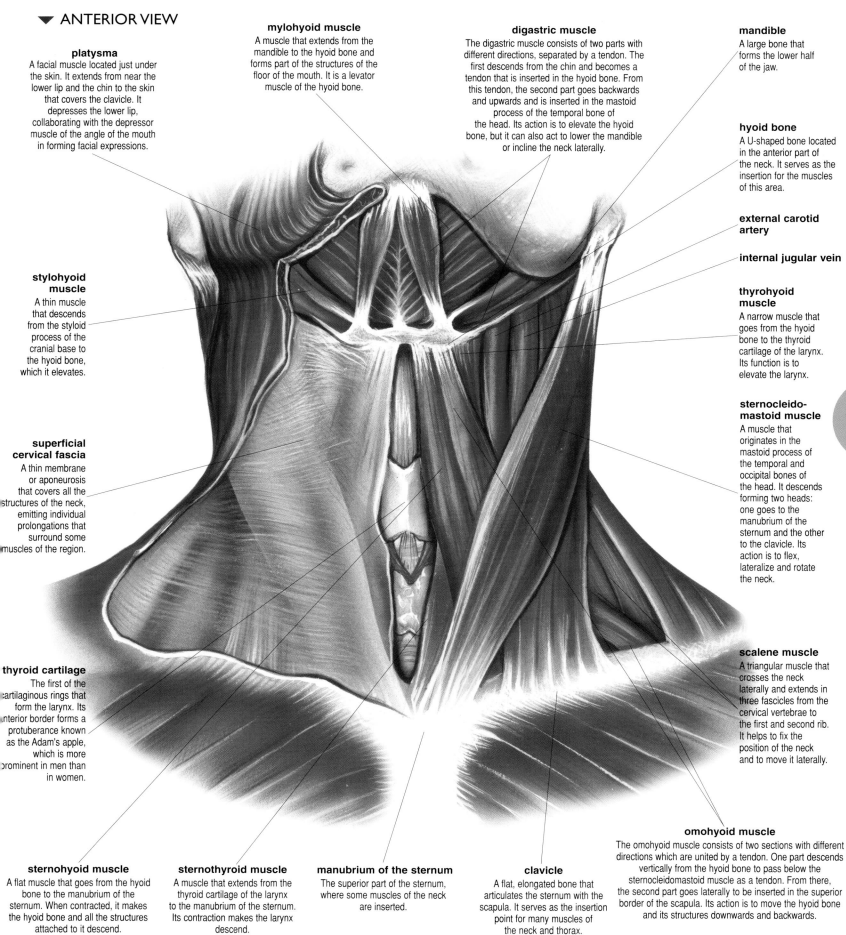

platysma
A facial muscle located just under the skin. It extends from near the lower lip and the chin to the skin that covers the clavicle. It depresses the lower lip, collaborating with the depressor muscle of the angle of the mouth in forming facial expressions.

mylohyoid muscle
A muscle that extends from the mandible to the hyoid bone and forms part of the structures of the floor of the mouth. It is a levator muscle of the hyoid bone.

digastric muscle
The digastric muscle consists of two parts with different directions, separated by a tendon. The first descends from the chin and becomes a tendon that is inserted in the hyoid bone. From this tendon, the second part goes backwards and upwards and is inserted in the mastoid process of the temporal bone of the head. Its action is to elevate the hyoid bone, but it can also act to lower the mandible or incline the neck laterally.

mandible
A large bone that forms the lower half of the jaw.

hyoid bone
A U-shaped bone located in the anterior part of the neck. It serves as the insertion for the muscles of this area.

external carotid artery

internal jugular vein

thyrohyoid muscle
A narrow muscle that goes from the hyoid bone to the thyroid cartilage of the larynx. Its function is to elevate the larynx.

stylohyoid muscle
A thin muscle that descends from the styloid process of the cranial base to the hyoid bone, which it elevates.

superficial cervical fascia
A thin membrane or aponeurosis that covers all the structures of the neck, emitting individual prolongations that surround some muscles of the region.

sternocleido-mastoid muscle
A muscle that originates in the mastoid process of the temporal and occipital bones of the head. It descends forming two heads: one goes to the manubrium of the sternum and the other to the clavicle. Its action is to flex, lateralize and rotate the neck.

29

thyroid cartilage
The first of the cartilaginous rings that form the larynx. Its anterior border forms a protuberance known as the Adam's apple, which is more prominent in men than in women.

scalene muscle
A triangular muscle that crosses the neck laterally and extends in three fascicles from the cervical vertebrae to the first and second rib. It helps to fix the position of the neck and to move it laterally.

omohyoid muscle
The omohyoid muscle consists of two sections with different directions which are united by a tendon. One part descends vertically from the hyoid bone to pass below the sternocleidomastoid muscle as a tendon. From there, the second part goes laterally to be inserted in the superior border of the scapula. Its action is to move the hyoid bone and its structures downwards and backwards.

sternohyoid muscle
A flat muscle that goes from the hyoid bone to the manubrium of the sternum. When contracted, it makes the hyoid bone and all the structures attached to it descend.

sternothyroid muscle
A muscle that extends from the thyroid cartilage of the larynx to the manubrium of the sternum. Its contraction makes the larynx descend.

manubrium of the sternum
The superior part of the sternum, where some muscles of the neck are inserted.

clavicle
A flat, elongated bone that articulates the sternum with the scapula. It serves as the insertion point for many muscles of the neck and thorax.

THE THORAX

▼ ANTERIOR VIEW

pectoralis minor muscle
A flat muscle located below the pectoralis major muscle. It originates in the third, fourth and fifth ribs and ascends obliquely. Its insertion is in the coracoid process of the scapula. When contracted, it depresses the scapula and thus all the shoulder. In addition it can elevate the ribs, becoming an inspiratory muscle.

subclavian muscle
A small muscle that ascends obliquely from the first costal cartilage to the inferior border of the clavicle. Its action is to make the clavicle, and thus the shoulder, descend.

pectoralis major muscle
A very wide triangular muscle that originates in the anterior aspect of the sternum, the clavicle and the last ribs. It converges outwards and is inserted by a tendon in the greater tubercle of the humerus. When contracted it lowers the arm when it is raised and, if it is already lowered, moves the shoulder forwards, bending the back. In addition it can elevate the thoracic cavity. It is innervated by the pectoral nerves.

intercostal muscles
Flat muscles located between the ribs, from the inferior border of the highest rib to the superior border of last rib. They consist of three layers of muscles: the internal, medial and external intercostals. Their action is to approximate the ribs to each other, widening or narrowing the chest as necessary during breathing.

serratus anterior muscle
A muscle located in the lateral wall of the thorax. It is formed of a series of heads that go from the nine or ten first ribs to the internal border of the scapula, bordering the thoracic wall laterally. When contracted it moves the internal border of the scapula forwards, elevating the shoulder. In addition it has inspiratory functions, elevating the ribs and widening the thorax.

aponeurotic sheath of the rectus abdominis muscle
An aponeurotic sheath that covers the rectus abdominis muscle. Its internal border joins with the border of the contralateral muscle to form the white line.

white line
A membrane that joins the aponeurotic sheaths that cover the superficial abdominal muscles. It marks the median line of the abdominal wall vertically.

rectus abdominis muscle
A flat muscle located in the anterior wall of the abdomen, to either side of the white line. It originates in the costal cartilages of the fifth, sixth and seventh ribs and in the xiphoid appendix of the sternum. It descends vertically and is inserted in the superior border of the pubis. When contracted it flexes the thorax forwards or elevates the pelvis, while simultaneously compressing the abdominal organs. It plays an important role in defecation and, in women, childbirth.

external oblique muscle of the abdomen
A wide muscle located in the lateral wall of the abdomen. It originates in the lower ribs and extends obliquely in the form of a fan formed by several fascicles that terminate in a tendinous membrane that merges with the sheath of the rectus abdominis muscle. Its contraction makes the ribs descend, flexes the thorax over the pelvis and inclines the thorax laterally.

30

THE THORAX

▼ POSTERIOR VIEW

deltoid muscle
A voluminous muscle that occupies all the superficial area of the shoulder. It originates inserted in the clavicle and the scapula. It descends to become a tendon that is inserted in the external face of the humerus. Its action is to elevate the arm to the horizontal and also to move it backwards and forwards.

trapezius muscle
A very wide triangular muscle that covers almost all the other muscles of the nape of the neck and a large part of the back. It originates in the occipital bone and the spinous processes of the cervical and dorsal vertebrae, and from there it converges on the shoulder, where it is inserted in the scapula and the clavicle. Its action is to elevate the shoulder and to incline the head sideways.

rhomboideus major muscle
A wide muscle that extends from the spinous processes of the first dorsal vertebrae to the internal border of the scapula. It acts to move the scapula inwards while inclining it.

rhomboideus minor muscle
A muscle located above the rhomboideus major muscle. It originates in the spinous processes of the last cervical vertebrae. It descends obliquely to be inserted in the internal border of the scapula. When contracted, it tilts the scapula and thus depresses the shoulder.

levator scapulae muscle
A triangular muscle that originates in the transverse processes of the four or five first cervical vertebrae. It converges to be inserted in the medial border of the scapula. It acts to incline the scapula and depress the shoulder, and also contributes to the lateral inclination of the head.

longissimus dorsi muscle
A muscle that originates in the common muscular mass of the erectors of the vertebral column. It ascends and is inserted in the transverse processes of the lumbar vertebrae and in the inferior border of the ribs. From there it sends a prolongation to the last cervical vertebrae that is called the longissimus muscle of the neck. It is an extensor muscle of the vertebral column which, like the iliocostalis muscle, fixes and maintains the column erect.

supraspinatus muscle
A triangular muscle that originates in the supraspinous fossa of the posterior face of the scapula. It terminates in a tendon which is inserted in the trochlea of the head of the humerus. It acts as a levator muscle of the arm, and also contributes slightly to the internal rotation of the arm.

infraspinatus fascia
A membranous layer that covers the infraspinous muscle.

infraspinatus muscle

latissimus dorsi muscle
A very wide, thin muscle that extends across the inferior area of the back. The internal part originates in the spinous processes of the lumbar and the dorsal vertebrae. The inferior part originates in the sacrum and the iliac crest and the superior part in the last three or four ribs. The muscle ascends towards the axilla and is inserted through a tendon in the humerus. With the arm raised, its contraction makes the humerus descend while rotating it internally. It also acts to elevate the ribs.

teres major muscle
A muscle that extends from the vertex and external border of the scapula to the humerus. Its action is to move the arm inwards and backwards. In addition it tilts the scapula, acting as an elevating muscle of the shoulder.

spinalis muscle
A muscle that originates in the erector spinae muscle group and ascends attached to the vertebral column to be inserted in the spinous processes of the lumbar and dorsal vertebrae. It continues towards the neck as the spinalis cervicis muscle. When contracted it extends the vertebral column.

iliocostalis muscle
A long muscle that crosses the back parallel to the vertebral column. It originates in the erector spinae muscle group and ascends to be inserted in each of the ribs. It terminates in the transverse processes of the last cervical vertebrae. The iliocostalis muscle is an extensor muscle of the vertebral column that also inclines the column laterally while fixing and maintaining it upright.

serratus posterior (inferior) muscle
A quadrilateral-shaped muscle located below the wide dorsal muscle. It is inserted in the spinous processes of the last dorsal vertebrae and first lumbar vertebrae. It ascends as four stepped heads that are inserted in the inferior borders of the four last ribs. It is an inspiratory muscle that makes the last ribs descend and widens the thorax.

intercostal muscles
Flat muscles located between the ribs, from the inferior border of the highest rib to the superior border of last rib. They consist of three layers of muscles; the internal, medial and external intercostals. Their action is to approximate the ribs to each other, widening or narrowing the chest as necessary during breathing.

serratus anterior muscle
A muscle located in the lateral wall of the thorax. It is formed of a series of fascicles that go from the nine or ten first ribs to the internal border of the scapula, bordering the thoracic wall laterally. When contracted it moves the internal border of the scapula forwards, elevating the shoulder. In addition it has inspiratory functions, elevating the ribs and widening the thorax.

31

THE ABDOMEN

▼ MALE ANTERIOR VIEW

pectoralis major muscle
A very wide triangular muscle, whose internal side originates in the anterior face of the sternum, the clavicle and the last ribs. It converges outwards and is inserted by a tendon in the greater tubercle of the humerus. When contracted it lowers the arm when it is raised and, if it is already lowered, moves the shoulder forwards, bending the back. In addition it can elevate the thoracic cavity. It is innervated by the pectoral nerves.

serratus anterior muscle
A muscle located in the lateral wall of the thorax. It is formed of a series of fascicles that go from the nine or ten first ribs to the internal border of the scapula, bordering the thoracic wall laterally. When contracted it moves the internal border of the scapula forwards, elevating the shoulder. In addition it has inspiratory functions, elevating the ribs and widening the thorax.

external oblique muscle of the abdomen
A wide muscle located in the lateral wall of the abdomen. It originates in the last ribs and extends obliquely in the form of a fan formed by several fascicles which terminate in a tendinous membrane that merges with the sheath of the rectus abdominis muscle. Its contraction makes the ribs descend, flexes the thorax over the pelvis and inclines the thorax laterally while compressing the organs of the abdominal cavity.

intercostal muscles
Flat muscles located between the ribs, from the inferior border of the highest rib to the superior border of the last rib. They consist of three layers of muscles: the internal, medial and external intercostals. Their action is to approximate the ribs to each other, widening or narrowing the chest as necessary during the action of breathing.

rectus abdominis muscle
A flat muscle located in the anterior face of the abdomen, to either side of the white line. It originates in the costal cartilages of the fifth, sixth and seventh ribs and in the xiphoid appendix of the sternum. It descends vertically and is inserted in the superior border of the pubis. When contracted, it flexes the thorax forwards or elevates the pelvis, while simultaneously compressing the abdominal organs. It plays an important role in defecation and, in women, childbirth.

32

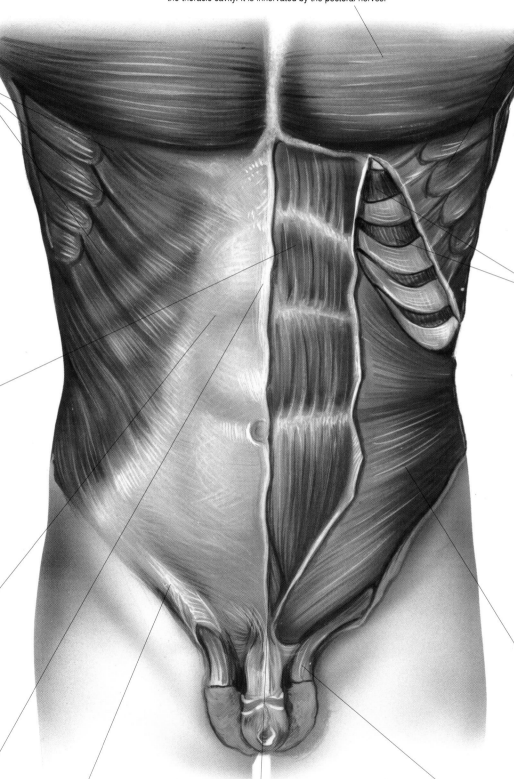

internal oblique muscle of the abdomen
A muscle located below the external oblique muscle. It originates in the anterosuperior iliac spine and the aponeurosis of the latissimus dorsi muscle and extends forwards like a fan. Superiorly it is inserted in the cartilages of the last ribs, inferiorly in the pubis, and medially it terminates in a wide membrane that merges with the sheath of the rectus abdominis muscle. Its action is to lower the ribs, to flex the thorax or to incline it laterally and to compress the abdominal organs. Below this muscle, the transverse muscle of the abdomen follows a parallel path.

aponeurotic sheath of the rectus abdominis muscle
An aponeurotic sheath that covers the rectus abdominis muscle. Its internal border joins with the border of the contralateral muscle to form the white line.

white line
A membrane that joins the aponeurotic sheaths that cover the superficial abdominal muscles. It marks the median line of the abdominal wall vertically, from the xiphoid process of the sterum to the pubis.

inguinal canal
A space located between the aponeurosis of the muscles of the inferointernal area of the abdomen. The inguinal canal is occupied by the spermatic cord in men and the round ligament in women.

pyramidalis muscle
A small, rudimentary muscle, whose function is not well defined. It is located in the inferior part of the abdomen, in front of the rectus abdominis muscle. It originates in the superior border of the pubis and extends obliquely upwards to reach the white line.

spermatic cord
A cord-like organ that contains the structures that connect with the testes, including the deferent duct, blood vessels and nerves.

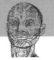

THE ABDOMEN

▼ MALE POSTERIOR VIEW

internal oblique muscle of the abdomen

A muscle located below the external oblique muscle. It originates in the anterosuperior iliac spine and the aponeurosis of the latissimus dorsi muscle. It extends forwards like a fan. Superiorly it is inserted in the cartilages of the last ribs, inferiorly in the pubis, and medially it terminates in a wide membrane that merges with the sheath of the rectus abdominis muscle. Its action is to lower the ribs, to flex the thorax or to incline it laterally and to compress the abdominal organs.

dorsolumbar fascia

A thick aponeurotic membrane that covers the muscles of the vertebral canal.

external oblique muscle of the abdomen

A wide muscle located in the lateral wall of the abdomen. It originates in the last ribs and extends obliquely in the shape of a fan formed by several fascicles that terminate in a tendinous membrane that merges with the sheath of the rectus abdominis muscle. Its contraction makes the ribs descend, flexes the thorax over the pelvis and inclines the thorax laterally while simultaneously compressing the organs of the abdominal cavity.

gluteus medius muscle

A very wide, thick muscle located below the gluteus maximus muscle. It originates in the iliac crest, the anterosuperior iliac spine, the external iliac fossa, the sacroiliac fibrous arch and the aponeurosis gluteus. It converges to be inserted in the greater trochanter of the femur. Its action is to raise the thigh in abduction or separation, while rotating it inwards and outwards. It is innervated by the superior gluteus nerve.

erector spinae muscle group

A powerful muscular mass that originates in the spinal aponeurosis and iliac crest. It ascends in ramifications that include the iliocostalis muscle, the longissimus dorsi muscle and the spinalis muscle.

gluteus minimus muscle

A muscle located beneath the gluteus medius muscle. It originates in the anterior part of the iliac crest and the external iliac fossa and is inserted in the greater trochanter of the femur. Its action is similar to that of the gluteus medius muscle, separating and rotating the thigh.

femoral aponeurosis or fascia lata

An aponeurotic sheath that covers and surrounds the muscles of the thigh. It extends from the pelvic area to the knee.

piriformis muscle

A triangular muscle that originates in the anterior face of the sacrum and is inserted in the greater trochanter of the femur. It crosses the greater sciatic notch to leave the pelvis. Its contraction rotates the thigh outwards. When the thigh is flexed over the pelvis, as occurs in the seated position, the muscle abducts or separates the thigh.

gluteus maximus muscle

A thick muscle that corresponds to the buttocks. It originates in the iliac crest of the ilium, the sacrum, the coccyx and the lumbodorsal fascia. It descends obliquely as a large muscular mass that is inserted in the iliotibial tracts and the gluteal tuberosity presented by the femur below the greater trochanter. One part merges with the tensor muscle of the fascia lata. Its main action is to extend the thigh backwards while rotating it outwards. It also helps to maintain the body upright by fixing the pelvis over the femur.

superior gemellus muscle

A flat muscle that originates in the sciatic spine of the iliac bone and from there goes outwards horizontally. It merges with the internal obturator muscle and the inferior gemellus muscle in a terminal tendon that is inserted in the greater trochanter of the femur. Its action is to rotate the thigh outwards.

inferior gemellus muscle

A flat muscle that originates in the tuberosity of the ischium and extends outwards to merge with the superior gemellus and the internal obturator muscles, to form a terminal tendon that is inserted in the greater trochanter of the femur. Its action is similar to that of the two muscles to which it is united, rotating the thigh outwards.

quadratus femoris muscle

A square muscle located in the posterior part of the hip joint. It originates in the tuberosity of the ischium and is inserted in the posterior border of the femur. Its action is to rotate the thigh outwards.

internal obturator muscle

A muscle that follows a passage parallel to the two gemelli muscles, which it lies between. It originates in the obturator membrane that covers the obturator foramen of the pelvis and in the bone ischium and pubis. It terminates with the superior and inferior gemellus muscles in a common tendon which is inserted in the greater trochanter of the femur. When contracted it rotates the thigh outwards.

spinal aponeurosis

A strong, pearly-coloured rhomboid membrane that is attached to the iliac crests and the sacrum and serves as the inferior insertion point for the iliocostalis and longissimus dorsi muscles.

33

DIAPHRAGM

▼ SUPERIOR VIEW

lumbar vertebrae
The first lumbar vertebrae serve as the insertion points for the tendons that are the terminations of the posterior part of the diaphragm muscle and its transverse processes.

spinal cord
Part of the nervous system which runs down the spine and is protected by the vertebrae. It is the origin of the spinal nerves.

intervertebral disc
A cartilaginous disc located between the bodies of the vertebrae. Its function is to cushion the pressures that can be transmitted from one vertebra to another.

pleura
A membrane that covers the lungs that are attached to the dome of the diaphragm.

DIAPHRAGM MUSCLE
A flat muscle that separates the thoracic and abdominal cavities. It is shaped like a concave vault. The diaphragm muscle is inserted posteriorly in the first lumbar vertebrae and the last ribs and anteriorly in the xiphoid process of the sternum and the last ribs.

azygos vein
A vein that ascends together with the vertebral bodies and joins the superior vena cava in the superior part of the thorax. In its course it collects the blood coming from the intercostal veins.

thoracic aorta
A large, artery that originates in the heart and crosses the thorax vertically, with branches that supply the thoracic organs. When it crosses the diaphragm to the abdomen it becomes the *abdominal aorta*.

intercostal muscles
Flat muscles located between the ribs, from the inferior border of the highest rib to the superior border of the last rib. They consist of three layers of muscles: the internal, medial and external intercostals. Their action is to approximate the ribs to each other, widening or narrowing the chest as necessary during breathing.

oesophagus
A tubular duct forming part of the alimentary canal. It connects the pharynx with the stomach after crossing the diaphragm.

pericardium
A saccular membrane that covers the heart and adheres to the dome of the diaphragm.

ribs
The last ribs serve as the insertion points for the diaphragmatic muscle and some muscles of the abdominal walls.

inferior vena cava
A large vein that collects the blood from the inferior extremities and the abdomen and carries it to the heart. As it ascends, it crosses the diaphragm.

sternum
A flat bone located in the anterior wall of the thorax, in whose lateral borders the ribs are united to close the thoracic cavity.

34

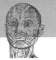

DIAPHRAGM

▼ INFERIOR VIEW

hiatus of the vena cava
An orifice located near the phrenic centre, through which the inferior vena cava passes from the abdomen to the thorax.

oesophageal hiatus
An orifice located in the centre of the diaphragm, through which the oesophagus passes from the thorax to the abdomen.

aortic hiatus
An orifice located under the median arcuate ligament, between the crus, through which the aorta passes from the thorax to the abdomen.

DIAPHRAGM MUSCLE
A flat muscle that separates the thoracic and abdominal cavities. It is shaped like a concave vault. The diaphragm muscle is inserted posteriorly in the first lumbar vertebrae, and the last ribs, and anteriorly in the xiphoid process of the sternum and the last ribs.

median arcuate ligament
A ligament that unites the crus of the diaphragm, leaving an orifice through which the aorta passes from the thorax to the abdomen.

crus of the diaphragm
The left and right crus are formed of muscle and tendon and are located in the posterior part of the diaphragm, which they attach to the bodies of the first lumbar vertebrae.

lateral arcuate ligament
A ligament in the form of an arch which unites the transverse process of the first lumbar vertebra with the twelfth rib. The quadratus lumborum passes under the ligament.

quadratus lumborum muscle
A flat muscle that extends vertically over the posterior surface of the abdomen, from the last rib to the iliac crest, and is inserted in the transverse processes of the lumbar vertebrae. Its action is to incline the vertebral column laterally.

psoas major muscle
A long muscle that crosses all the posterior surface of the abdomen. It originates in the last rib and leaves the pelvic cavity to be inserted in the smaller trochanter of the femur. When contracted it flexes the thigh and inclines the vertebral column forwards or laterally.

medial arcuate ligament
A ligament that forms an arch between the posterior pillar of the diaphragm and the transverse process of the first lumbar vertebra. The psoas major muscle passes under the ligament.

transverse muscle of the abdomen
A muscle that crosses the lateral wall of the abdomen transversally, from the transverse processes of the lumbar vertebrae and the iliac crest to the anterior face, where it merges with a wide membrane that covers the other muscles of the anterior face.

35

THE MALE PERINEUM

bulbocavernosus muscle
An erector muscle that originates in the prerectal area and goes upwards and forwards, bordering the spongy portion of the urethra and terminating in the cavernous bodies of the penis.

penis
The male genital organ. It contains internal cavernous bodies which fill with blood during sexual arousal and erect the penis. The penis carries the male urethra through which both semen and urine are expelled.

ischiocavernosus muscle
A muscle that goes from the cavernous bodies of the penis to the ischium. Its action is to facilitate the entrance of blood in the penile cavernous bodies and to provoke the erection of the penis.

deep fascia of the penis
A cylindrical, membranous sheath that surrounds the cavernous bodies of the penis.

superficial transverse muscle of perineum
A small muscle that goes from the bone ischium towards the median line, and is inserted in the prerectal raphe. The deep transverse muscle of the perineum follows a parallel course. Its action is complementary to that of the levator muscle of the anus, contributing to the process of defecation. It also intervenes in urination and ejaculation.

prerectal raphe
A membrane that unites the anterior part of the anus with the base of the penis.

36

ischiococcygeus muscle
A flat, triangular muscle located behind the levator muscle of the anus. It is inserted anteriorly in the sciatic spine and extends to the coccyx. Its action is to support the intrapelvic organs.

anus
The external opening of the rectum through which the faecal matter is expelled.

gluteus maximus muscle
A thick muscle that corresponds to the buttocks. It extends the iliac crest, the sacrum, the coccyx and the aponeurosis and ligaments of the area, to the femur. Its action is to extend the thigh backwards, to rotate it outwards and fix the pelvis in the upright position.

termination of the coccyx
The last coccygeal vertebrae that are covered by an aponeureosis and serve as the insertion for various muscles of the region.

external anal sphincter
A ring-shaped muscle that surrounds the anal orifice, which has prolongations to the skin of the perineum and the anococcygeal raphe. It acts as a sphincter, impeding defecation when contracted, and relaxing to allow faecal matter to pass.

levator muscle of the anus
A flat muscle that arises from the pubic bone to the rectum and the anus, passing by the lateral wall of the prostate. It has two parts, one superficial and another deep. It contributes to the act of defecation by compressing the rectum and elevating the anus, and also supports the intrapelvic organs.

THE FEMALE PERINEUM

gracilis muscle
A muscle of the leg, not the perineum. It crosses the internal part of the thigh, from the pubis to the femur. Its action is to flex the thigh.

ischiocavernosus muscle
A muscle that goes from the pelvis to the base of the clitoris. Its action is to facilitate the entrance of blood to the cavernous bodies of the clitoris and to provoke its erection.

clitoris
An erectile organ located in the vertex of union of the two labia majora. It is formed of cavernous tissue that fills with blood during sexual arousal.

urethral orifice
A small orifice located below the clitoris and above the vaginal orifice which is the termination of the urethra where the urine is expelled.

bulbocavernosus muscle
A muscle that originates in the anterior region of the anus and extends forwards to the distal area of the vagina and the urethra, reaching the base of the clitoris. It acts to facilitate the erection of the clitoris and vaginal contraction and the secretion of the mucous glands during intercourse.

labia minora
Mucocutaneous folds that border the vaginal orifice laterally.

vaginal orifice
An orifice that joins the vagina and the vulva and which is located below the urethral ostium. It receives the penis during intercourse and acts as the birth canal.

superficial transverse muscle of perineum
A small muscle that goes from the ischium to the prerectal raphe. Its action is complementary to that of the levator muscle of the anus, contributing to the process of defecation.

perineal raphe
A membrane that unites the posterior part of the vaginal orifice with the anterior part of the anus, below the perineum.

ischiococcygeus muscle
A flat, triangular muscle located behind the levator muscle of the anus. It is inserted anteriorly in the sciatic spine and extends to the coccyx. Its action is to support the intrapelvic organs.

anus
The external opening of the rectum through which the faecal matter is expelled.

gluteus maximus muscle
The gluteus maximus is a muscle of the pelvis, not the perineum. It goes from the coccyx, the sacrum and the iliac crests to the femur. Its action is fundamental for walking and the stability of the pelvis.

levator muscle of the anus
A flat muscle that goes from the pubic bone to the rectum and the anus. It consists of two fascicles, one superficial and another deep. It contributes to the act of defecation by compressing the rectum and elevating the anus, and also supports the intrapelvic organs.

external anal sphincter
A ring-shaped muscle that surrounds the anal orifice. It acts as a sphincter, impeding defecation when contracted, and relaxing to allow it.

termination of the coccyx
The last coccygeal vertebrae that are covered by an aponeureosis and serve as the insertion for various muscles of the region.

anococcygeal ligament
A membrane that extends from the posterior border of the anus to the last vertebrae of the coccyx.

37

THE SHOULDER AND ARM. SUPERFICIAL MUSCLES

▼ ANTERIOR VIEW

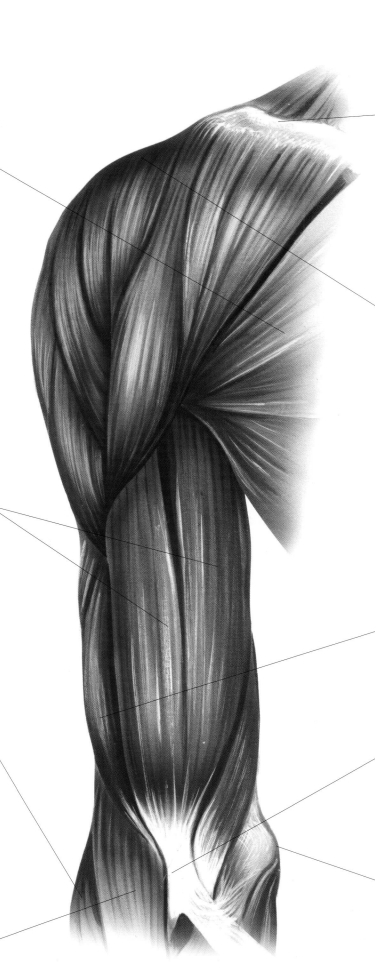

clavicle
An elongated bone that joins the sternum with the scapula. It is the insertion for various muscles of the neck, shoulder and pectoral area.

pectoralis major muscle
A very wide triangular muscle, whose internal side is inserted in the anterior face of the sternum, the clavicle and the last ribs. It converges outwards and is inserted by a tendon in the greater tubercle of the humerus. When contracted, it lowers the arm when it is raised and, if it is already lowered, moves the shoulder forwards, bending the back. In addition it can elevate the thoracic cavity. It is innervated by the pectoral nerves.

deltoid muscle
A voluminous muscle that occupies all the superficial area of the shoulder. It is inserted in the clavicle and the scapula. It descends to become a tendon that is inserted in the external face of the humerus. Its action is to elevate the arm to the horizontal and also to move it backwards and forwards.

38

biceps brachii muscle
A thick muscle that occupies the anterior face of the arm. It consists of two parts: an external or a long portion that originates in the external angle of the scapula, and a short internal portion that originates in the coracoid process of the scapula. The two portions merge to form a single muscular mass that becomes a tendon which crosses the elbow and is inserted in the head of the radius. The biceps muscle flexes the forearm on the arm, places it in supination or external rotation and elevates the arm.

músculo braquial anterior
Músculo muy ancho que se sitúa por debajo del bíceps braquial y sobresale por su lado. Se inserta en la cara interna y externa del húmero; desde allí sus fibras descienden, cruzan el codo por su parte anterior y se fijan en el hueso cúbito. Su principal acción es doblar el antebrazo sobre el brazo.

extensor carpi radialis longus
A flat muscle that is located below the brachioradialis muscle. It originates in the external border of the humerus, crosses the external border of the forearm and terminates as a tendon that crosses the wrist joint and is inserted in the base of the second metacarpal bone of the hand. When contracted, it extends the second metacarpal bone, moving the hand in extension over the forearm.

brachialis muscle
A very wide muscle that is located below the biceps muscle. It originates in the internal and external faces of the humerus, from where it descends crossing the anterior part of the elbow to be inserted in the ulna. Its main action is to double the forearm over the arm.

epicondyle
A bony protuberance located in the internal area of the inferior extremity of the humerus, where ligaments of the elbow joint and muscles of the forearm are inserted.

brachioradialis muscle
A muscle that originates in the external border of the humerus and, after crossing all the forearm, forms a tendon that is inserted in the inferior end of the radius. Its main action is to flex the forearm on the arm.

THE SHOULDER AND ARM. SUPERFICIAL MUSCLES

▼ POSTERIOR VIEW

trapezius muscle
A very wide triangular muscle that covers almost all the other muscles of the nape of the neck and a large part of the back. It originates in the external protuberance of the occipital bone and the spinous processes of the seven cervical and twelve dorsal vertebrae. The vertex of the triangle is located in the shoulder where the trapezius is inserted in the acromion and spine of the scapula and the clavicle. Its action is to elevate the shoulder and to incline the head sideways.

**spine
of the scapula**
An elevated protuberance located in the posterior face of the scapula, which serves as the insertion of the deltoid and trapezius muscles.

infraspinatus fascia
A membranous layer that covers the infraspinous muscle. It occupies almost all the posterior face of the scapula and extends to the head of the humerus where it is inserted.

tendon of triceps brachii
The three muscle heads that form the brachial triceps become a tendon that reaches the elbow and is inserted in the olecranon of the ulna.

deltoid muscle
A voluminous muscle that occupies all the superficial area of the shoulder. It is inserted in the clavicle and the scapula. It descends to become a tendon that is inserted in the external face of the humerus. Its action is to elevate the arm to the horizontal and also to move it backwards and forwards.

teres major muscle
A muscle that extends from the vertex and external border of the scapula to the humerus. Its action is to move the arm inwards and backwards. In addition it tilts the scapula, acting as an elevating muscle of the shoulder.

triceps brachii muscle
A thick muscle that occupies the posterior area of the arm. Its superior part consists of three portions: the long portion, which originates in the external border of the scapula, the external portion or vastus externus, which originates in the posterior face of the humerus, and the internal portion or vastus medialis muscle that originates in the posterointernal face of the humerus. The three portions unite to form a thick muscular mass that terminates in a tendon that is inserted in the olecranon of the ulna. The triceps brachii is an extensor of the forearm over the arm.

latissimus dorsi muscle
A very wide, thin muscle that extends across the inferior area of the back. The internal part is inserted in the spinous processes of the lumbar vertebrae and the dorsal vertebrae. The inferior part is inserted in the sacrum and the iliac crest and the superior part in the last three or four ribs. The muscle ascends towards the axilla and is inserted through a tendon in the humerus. With the arm raised, its contraction makes the humerus descend while rotating it internally. It also acts to elevate the ribs.

brachioradialis muscle
A long muscle that extends along the external border of the forearm. It originates in the external border of the humerus and, after crossing all the forearm, converts a tendon that is inserted in the inferior end of the radius. Its main action is to flex the forearm over the arm, although it also rotates the forearm outwards when it is rotated inwards, or inwards when it is rotated outwards.

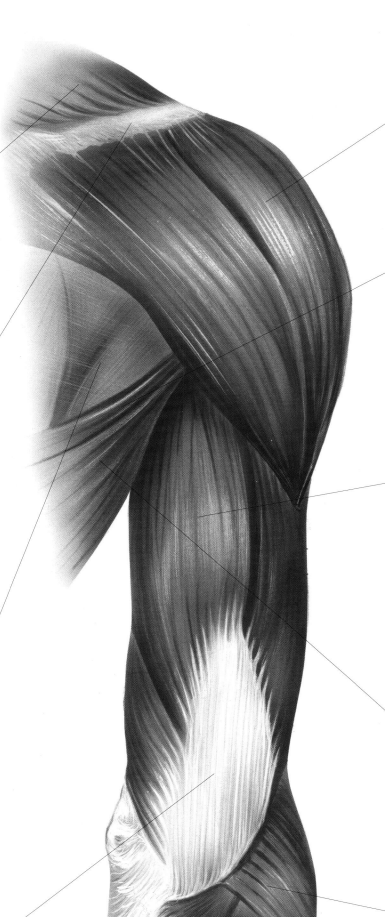

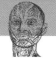

THE FOREARM. SUPERFICIAL MUSCLES

▼ ANTERIOR VIEW

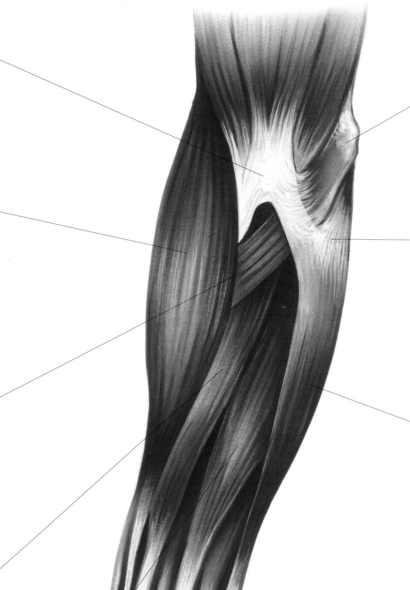

tendon of the biceps brachii muscle

brachioradialis muscle
A long muscle that extends along the external border of the forearm. It originates in the external border of the humerus and, after crossing all the forearm, converts to a tendon that is inserted in the inferior end of the radius. Its main action is to flex the forearm over the arm, although it also rotates the forearm outwards when it is rotated inwards, or inwards when it is rotated outwards.

pronator teres muscle
A flat muscle that extends obliquely from the epitrochlea of the humerus and the coronoid process of the ulna to the external face of the radius. It rotates the forearm inwards in pronation and also flexes the forearm over the arm.

flexor carpi radialis muscle
A muscle that crosses the anterior face of the forearm obliquely, from the epitrochlea of the humerus to the second metacarpal bone of the hand. When contracted, it flexes the hand on the forearm and the forearm on the arm. It also moves the hand outwards.

palmaris longus muscle
The flexor carpi radialis muscle follows a parallel passage to the palmaris longus, from the humeral epitrochlea to the anterior face of the annular ligament of the wrist and the palmar aponeurosis of the hand, where it is inserted by a long tendon. Its action is to flex the hand anteriorly on the forearm and to tense the palmar aponeurosis.

epicondyle
A bony protuberance located in the internal area of the inferior extremity of the humerus, where ligaments of the elbow joint and muscles of the forearm are inserted.

aponeurotic sheath of the forearm
A cylindrical sheath that totally covers the muscles of the forearm and the arm. In its internal superior part it is inserted in the epitrochlea of the humerus.

flexor carpi ulnaris muscle
A muscle that occupies the internal border of the forearm. It originates in the superior part of the epicondyle of the humerus and in the olecranon of the ulna. It descends along the internal border of the ulna, crosses the wrist joint and is inserted by a tendon into the carpus. It flexes the hand on the forearm, turning the palm outwards.

flexor digitorum superficialis muscle
A wide muscle that occupies almost all the medial plane of the anterior face of the forearm. It originates in the epitrochlea of the humerus and the coronoid process of the ulna. It forms a wide muscular mass which divides into four muscular fascicles that terminate in four tendons that cross the wrist joint below the annular ligament of the carpus. In the palm of the hand, they go to the second phalanges of the second, third, fourth and fifth fingers. Its action is to flex the second phalange of the fingers on the first, the fingers on the hand, the hand on the forearm and the forearm on the arm.

flexor retinaculum
A fibrous ligament that covers the anterior face of the carpus. It serves as the insertion for many muscles of the palm of the hand. The tendons of the muscles' flexors pass below the ligament to the palmar region.

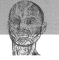

THE FOREARM. SUPERFICIAL MUSCLES

▼ POSTERIOR VIEW

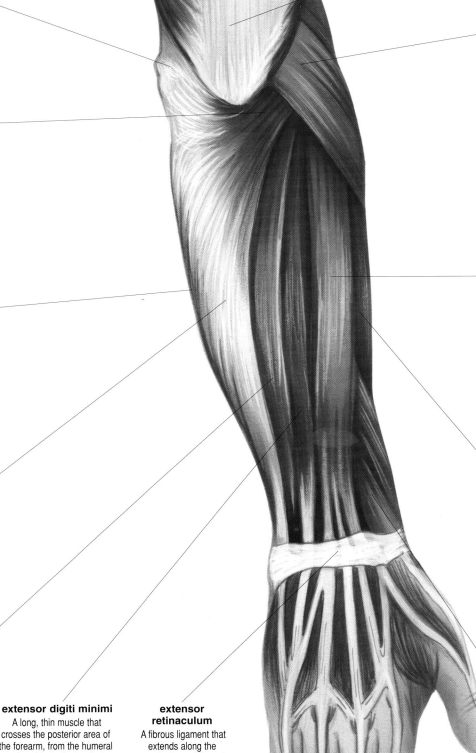

epicondyle
A bony protuberance located in the internal area of the inferior extremity of the humerus, where ligaments of the elbow joint and muscles of the forearm are inserted.

anconeus muscle
A flat, triangular muscle that originates in the epicondyle of the humerus and which extends to be inserted in the posterior border of the ulna. It collaborates with the brachial triceps muscle in extending the forearm over the arm.

flexor carpi ulnaris muscle
A muscle that occupies the internal border of the forearm. It originates in the superior part of the epicondyle of the humerus and in the olecranon of the ulna. It descends along the internal border of the ulna, crosses the wrist joint and is inserted by a tendon into the carpus. It flexes the hand on the forearm, turning the palm outwards.

aponeurotic sheath of the forearm
A cylindrical sheath that totally covers the muscles of the forearm and the arm. It is inserted, in its internal superior part, in the epitrochlea of the humerus.

extensor carpi ulnaris muscle
A muscle that extends obliquely across the posterior area of the forearm, from the epicondyle of the humerus, across the wrist joint, and terminates in the fifth metacarpal bone. When contracted, it doubles the hand backwards over the forearm in extension, while simultaneously inclining it inwards in adduction.

extensor digiti minimi
A long, thin muscle that crosses the posterior area of the forearm, from the humeral epicondyle to the two last phalanges of the fifth finger, where it is inserted by means of a tendon that merges in its terminal part with the tendon of the extensor digitorum muscle. Its action is to extend the fifth finger.

extensor retinaculum
A fibrous ligament that extends along the posterior face of the wrist joint. The tendons of the muscles of the posterior area of the forearm pass under this ligament to the hand.

tendon of the triceps brachii muscle

extensor carpi radialis longus
A flat muscle that is located below the brachiradialis muscle. It originates in the external border of the humerus, crosses the external border of the forearm and terminates as a tendon that crosses the wrist joint and is inserted in the base of the second metacarpal bone of the hand. When contracted it extends the second metacarpal bone, moving the hand in extension over the forearm.

extensor digitorum muscle
A flat muscle that originates in the epicondyle of the humerus. It descends and divides into three tendons, which cross under the extensor retinaculum and terminate in the second and third phalanges of the second, third, fourth and fifth fingers. Its action is to extend the third phalange over the second, the second over the first, the fingers over the hands, the hand over the forearm and the forearm over the arm.

extensor carpi radialis brevis
A muscle located in the external area of the forearm, below the extensor carpi radialis longus. It extends from the epicondyle of the humerus and the external lateral ligament of the elbow joint to the wrist joint and is inserted in the base of the third metacarpal bone. When contracted it turns the hand backwards over the forearm in extension.

abductor pollicis longus
A muscle that extends from the posterior face of the ulna and radius to the base of the first metacarpal bone, crossing the wrist joint under the posterior annular ligament. It turns the thumb outwards in abduction and also the rest of the hand, and rotates it.

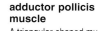

THE HAND. SUPERFICIAL MUSCLES

▼ ANTERIOR VIEW

opponens digiti minimi muscle
A muscle located below the short flexor and the separator of the fifth finger. It originates in the flexor retinaculum and is inserted in the fifth metacarpal bone. It moves the fifth finger forwards and towards the median line of the hand in opposition to the thumb.

palmar interosseal muscles
Small muscles located in the palmar fingers, in the spaces between the metacarpal bones where they originate. From there, they merge with the corresponding tendon of the extensor digitorum muscle of the second, fourth and fifth fingers. Their action is to flex the first phalanges and to extend the second and third, while at the same time approximating the four last fingers to each other. They are innervated by branches of the ulnar nerve.

tendons of the flexor digitorum profundis muscle
The tendons of this muscle, whose muscular mass is found in the deep area of the anterior part of the forearm, when they reach the level of first phalanges of the four last fingers, pass through a small opening created by the bifurcation of the tendons of the flexor digitorum superficialis muscle. They terminate in the third phalanges of the four last fingers. Their action is to flex the fingers over the hand and the hand over the forearm.

tendons of the flexor digitorum superficialis muscle
The tendons of the muscle divide into two at the level of the first phalanges of the fingers, leaving small openings through which the tendons of the flexor digitrum profundus. The two tendons are inserted in the lateral faces of the second phalanges. Their action is to flex the fingers over the hand and the hand over the arm.

flexor digiti minimi muscle
A muscle that follows a path parallel to the abductor digiti minimi muscle. It extends from the carpus and the flexor retinaculum to the base of the first phalange of the fifth finger, where it is inserted by a tendon that is common to the abductor digiti minimi muscle. Its action is to bend the first phalange of the fifth finger over the palm of the hand.

adductor pollicis muscle
A triangular-shaped muscle that consists of two origins: one oblique, in the carpal bones, and the other transverse, in the second and third metacarpal bones. The muscle bodies converge and are inserted in the first phalange of the thumb. It carries the thumb inwards, in a movement of approach or adduction.

flexor pollicis brevis muscle
A muscle located below the abductor or short separator of the thumb. It originates in the flexor retinaculum and the carpal bones and is inserted in the first phalanx of the thumb. Its action is to move the thumb forwards and inwards.

abductor digiti minimi
A muscle that occupies the internal border of the palm of the hand, from the carpus to the first phalange of the fifth finger. When contracted, it separates the fifth finger from the central axis of the hand and flexes the first phalange of the fifth finger over the palm of the hand.

abductor pollicis brevis muscle
A muscle located in the superficial area of the thenar eminence, which goes from the flexor retinaculum to the first phalanx of the thumb. When contracted, it separates or abducts the thumb outwards, while simultaneously moving it forwards.

flexor retinaculum
A fibrous ligament that covers the anterior face of the carpus. It serves as the insertion for many muscles of the palm of the hand. The tendons of the muscles' flexors pass below the ligament to the palmar region.

opponens pollicis muscle
A small triangular muscle that originates in the flexor retinaculum and inserts into the first metacarpal bone. When contracted, it carries the first metacarpal bone and the thumb forwards and inwards, while rotating it slightly internally, leaving the thumb in opposition to the other four fingers.

42

hypothenar eminence

thenar eminence

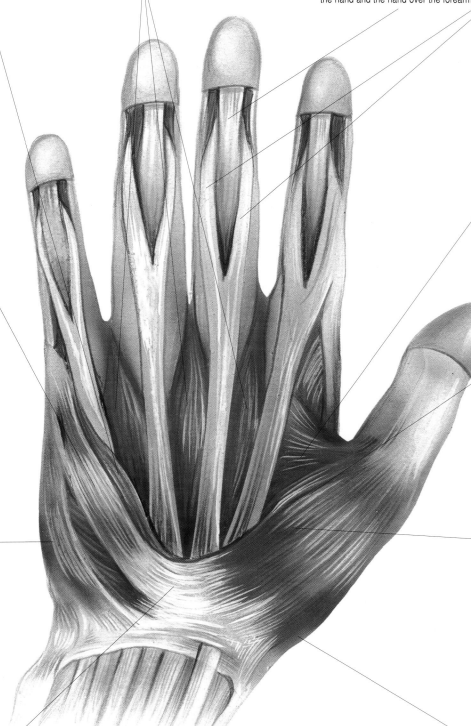

THE HAND. SUPERFICIAL MUSCLES

▼ POSTERIOR VIEW

tendons of the extensor digitorum muscle
The tendons of this muscle, whose muscular mass is in the posterior part of the forearm, are inserted into the phalanges of the second, third, fourth and fifth fingers. Their action is to extend the phalanges, the fingers and the hand.

tendons of the flexor digitorum superficialis muscle
The tendons of the muscle divide into two at the height of the first phalanx of the four last fingers, leaving small openings through which the tendons of the deep common flexor muscle pass. The two tendons are inserted in the lateral faces of the second phalanges. Their action is to flex the fingers over the hand and the hand over the arm.

dorsal interosseal muscles
Small muscles located on the dorsal surface of the hand in the spaces between the metacarpal bones where they originate. They descend to merge with the corresponding tendon of the extensor digitorum muscle of the second, fourth and fifth fingers. Their action is to flex the first phalanx and to extend the second and third phalanges while simultaneously separating the four last fingers.

tendon of the extensor pollicis brevis muscle
The tendon of this muscle, whose mass is in the deep area of the posterior face of the forearm. It reaches the first phalanx of the thumb and its action is to extend it.

tendon of the extensor pollicis longus muscle
The tendon of this muscle, whose mass is in the deep area of the posterior face of the forearm. It reaches the second phalanx of the thumb, and its action is to extend it.

tendon of the extensor digiti minimi
The tendon of this muscle, whose muscular mass is in the posterior part of the forearm merges with the extensor digitorum muscle to form a tendon which inserts into the fifth finger. Its action is to extend the fifth finger.

extensor retinaculum
A fibrous ligament that extends along the posterior surface of the carpus. The tendons of the extensor muscles pass under this ligament to the dorsum of the hand.

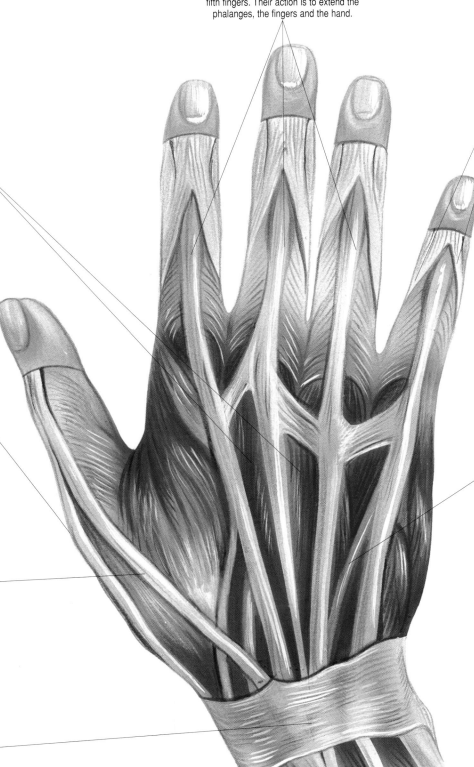

43

THE THIGH. SUPERFICIAL MUSCLES

▼ ANTERIOR VIEW

anterosuperior iliac spine
A bony protuberance that is the anterior limit of the iliac crest.

iliopsoas muscle
A muscle that consists of two parts: the psoas major, which originates in the last rib and the lumbar vertebrae, and the iliacus which originates in the ilium and the sacrum. The two parts join and when they reach the thigh they are inserted in the lesser trochanter of the femur. Its action is to double the thigh over the pelvis, to incline it forwards and fix it to the column in the upright position.

pectinate muscle
A flat muscle that joins the pelvis and the thigh. It originates in the pubic bone and the inguinal ligament, and descends obliquely to be inserted as a tendon in the lesser trochanter of the femur. When contracted, it approximates the thigh inwards in adduction, while simultaneously rotating the thigh outwards. It also collaborates in the flexion of the thigh over the pelvis.

tensor muscle of the fascia lata
A flat muscle that originates in the iliac crest and anterosuperior iliac spine and the aponeurosis of the gluteus muscles. It descends laterally with a fascicle that merges with the ligaments of the fascia lata or femoral aponeurosis, and other fascicles that terminate in the external tuberosity of the tibia. When contracted, it stretches the external part of the femoral aponeurosis, while simultaneously abducting or separating the thigh. It also helps to incline the pelvis to one side and fix it over the inferior extremities in the standing position.

pubic bone
The anterior bone of the three that form the hip bone. In this area it presents a crest or pectinate line, in which muscles of the thigh and the pelvis are inserted.

gracilis muscle
A long, thin muscle that originates in the pubic bone and follows the medial border of the thigh to reach the superior part of the tibia, where it is inserted by a tendon that is common to two other muscles, the semitendinosus and the sartorius. The tendon is known as the pes anserinus. The gracilis muscle is a flexor of the leg over the thigh and an approximator of the thigh.

44

sartorius muscle
A long, thin muscle that crosses the anterior surface of the thigh obliqely, from the anterosuperior iliac spine to the medial part of the superior extremity of the tibia, where it is inserted. In this area, it forms a thick tendon with the gracilis muscle and semitendinosus muscle, and is called the pes anserinus. When contracted, it bends the leg on the thigh and the thigh on the pelvis, while simultaneously rotating and separating the thigh externally.

adductor longus muscle
Also called the first adductor muscle. It extends from the pelvis to the thigh, and follows a parallel passage to the pectinate muscle. It originates in the pubic bone and is inserted in the medial border of the femur. Like the other adductor muscles, it approximates the thigh inwards and rotates it outwards.

quadriceps femoris muscle
A thick muscle that occupies the anterior face of the thigh. It is formed of four muscles: the vastus lateralis muscle, vastus medialis muscle, the rectus femoris muscle and the vastus intermedius muscle, which is in a deeper plane. These muscles finish in a wide common tendinous aponeurosis that is inserted in the patella and then descends as the patellar tendon, that terminates in the anterior tuberosity of the tibia. Its main action is to extend the leg over the thigh, although it also acts to double the thigh over the pelvis.

rectus femoris muscle
A portion of the quadriceps that occupies the central position. It originates in two tendons in the anteroinferior iliac spine and the articular capsule of the hip joint.

vastus lateralis muscle
The external portion of the four muscles that compose the quadriceps. It originates in the greater trochanter of the femur.

patellar ligament
A thick ligament that extends from the vertex of the patella to the anterior tuberosity of the tibia. It is a prolongation of the tendon of inferior insertion of the four portions of the quadriceps muscle.

patella
A flat, round bone that occupies the anterior face of the joint of the knee.

vastus medialis muscle
A part of the quadriceps muscle that is attached to the internal part of the femur. It originates in the area of transition between the body and the neck of this bone.

THE THIGH. SUPERFICIAL MUSCLES

▼ POSTERIOR VIEW

gluteus maximus muscle

A thick muscle that corresponds to the buttocks. It originates in the iliac crest of the ilium, the sacrum, the coccyx and the lumbodorsal fascia. It descends obliquely as a large muscular mass which is inserted in the iliotibial tracts and the gluteal tuberosity presented by the femur below the greater trochanter. One part merges with the tensor muscle of the fascia lata. Its main action is to extend the thigh backwards while rotating it outwards. It also helps to maintain the body upright by fixing the pelvis over the femur.

adductor magnus muscle

A wide muscle that extends from the ischium of the pelvis to the medial border of the femur. It is located below the sartorius, adductor minimis and quadriceps muscles of the anterior face of the thigh. Its action is to approximate the thigh inwards and to rotate it.

gracilis muscle

A long, thin muscle that originates in the pubic bone and follows the internal border of the thigh to reach the superior part of the tibia, where it is inserted by a tendon that is common to two other muscles, the semitendinosus and the sartorius. The tendon is known as the pes anserinus. The gracilis muscle is a flexor of the leg over the thigh and an approximator of the thigh.

semitendinosus muscle

A muscle that originates in the ischium, and descends along the posterior surface of the thigh. After passing the medial border of the knee, it becomes anterior and is converted into the tendon known as the pes anserinus, which serves as the common insertion in the superior extremity of the tibia for two other muscles: the sartorius and the gracilis muscles. When contracted, it doubles the leg over the thigh and rotates the thigh internally. It also acts as an extensor of the thigh over the pelvis.

thoracolumbar aponeurosis

A thick membrane that covers the musculature of the back and reaches the iliac crest of the pelvis.

semimembranous muscle

A muscle partially covered by the semitendinosus muscle. It is called the semimembranous muscle because its superior third is composed of a wide tendinous membrane. It originates in the ischium and is inserted in the superior extremity of the tibia. Its action is similar to the semitendinosus muscle.

gluteal aponeurosis

An extremely thick aponeurotic membrane that covers the gluteal musculature externally. It originates in the iliac crest and terminates in the thigh where it merges with the femoral fascia or fascia lata.

short head of the biceps femoris muscle

The short portion of the two that form the superior part of the biceps femoral muscle. It originates in the internal border of the femur, in the linea aspera.

iliotibial tract

A fibrous membrane that crosses the thigh laterally and superficially and is formed by the prolongation of the membrane that covers the thigh called the fascia lata.

biceps femoris muscle

A thick muscle that crosses the external part of the posterior thigh. The superior part is formed of two heads, the short and long heads, which merge and terminate in a single very long tendon that is inserted in the superior extremity of the fibula. The biceps femoral flexes the leg over the thigh, while simultaneously rotating the thigh slightly externally. It also acts as an extensor of the thigh over the pelvis.

long head of biceps femoris muscle

One of the two heads that form the biceps femoris muscle in its superior part. It originates in the ischium and descends obliquely down the posterior face of the thigh.

popliteal fossa

A rhomboidal space located in the dorsal face of the knee, which is framed by the muscles of the posterior face of the thigh and the leg (semimembranous, biceps femoris and gastrocnemius muscles). It gives passage to the blood vessels and the nerves going from the thigh to the leg.

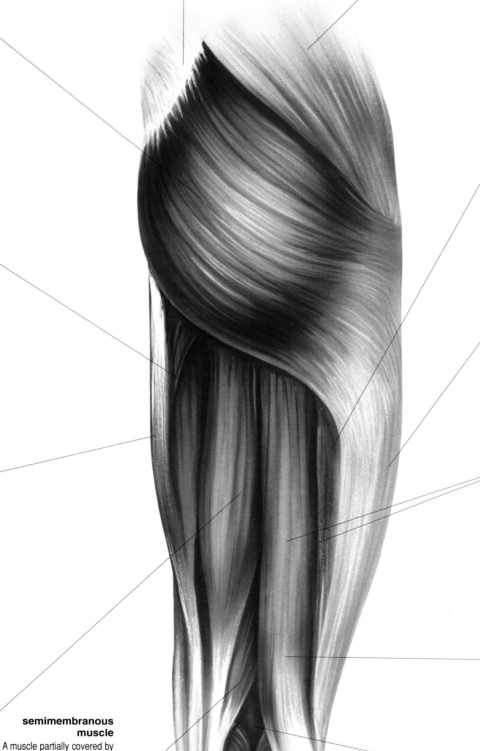

45

LEG. SUPERFICIAL MUSCLES

▼ ANTERIOR VIEW

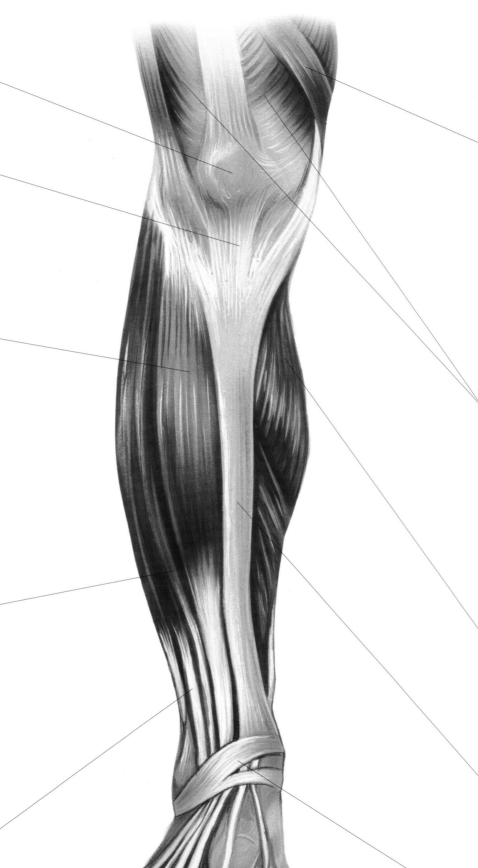

patella
A flat, round bone that occupies the anterior face of the joint of the knee.

patellar ligament
A thick ligament that extends from the vertex of the patella to the anterior tuberosity of the tibia. It is a prolongation of the tendon of inferior insertion of the four portions of the quadriceps muscle.

anterior tibial muscle
A voluminous muscle that crosses the anterior face of the leg to reach the internal border of the foot. It originates in the superior extremity of the tibia. It descends and converges to become a powerful tendon that passes below the extensor retinaculum and is inserted in the first metatarsal and the first cuneiform bone. When contracted, it flexes the foot over the leg, carries the foot towards the median line and rotates it inwards.

extensor digitorum longus muscle
A flat muscle that shares a common origin with the anterior tibial muscle and follows a parallel trajectory until reaching the dorsum of the foot, when it divides into four tendons that go to each of the four lateral toes, where they are inserted in the second and third phalanges. Its action is to extend the last four toes over the dorsal face of the foot, while simultaneously doubling the foot over the leg and

extensor hallucis longus muscle
A muscle that is partially covered by the tibial anterior and common extensor of the fingers' muscles. It originates in the fibula and the interosseal ligament and descends to the flexor retinaculum of the tarsus, which it passes beneath converted into a tendon. It follows the internal border of the dorsal part of the foot and is inserted in the first and second phalanges of the big toe. It is an extensor muscle of the big toe over the foot and also flexes or doubles the leg and turns it inwards.

sartorius muscle
A long, thin muscle that crosses the anterior surface of the thigh obliqely, from the anterosuperior iliac spine to the internal part of the superior extremity of the tibia, where it is inserted. In this area, it shares a thick tendon with the gracilis muscle and semitendinosus muscle, a tendon that receives the name of pes anserinus. When contracted, it doubles the leg on the thigh and the thigh on the pelvis, while simultaneously rotating and separating the thigh externally.

quadriceps femoris muscle
A thick muscle that occupies the anterior face of the thigh. It is formed of four fascicles: the vastus lateralis muscle, vastus medialis muscle, the rectus femoris muscle and the vastus intermedius muscle, which is in a deeper plane. These fascicles finish in a wide common tendinous aponeurosis that is inserted in the patella and then descends as the patellar tendon, that terminates in the anterior tuberosity of the tibia. Its main action is to extend the leg over the thigh, although it also acts to double the thigh over the pelvis.

medial gastrocnemius muscle
The medial portion of the gemellus or gastrocnemius muscle originates in the internal condyle of the femur. In the medial third of the leg it is united with the soleus to form the terminal part of a single muscle which is inserted in the Achilles tendon.

tibial crest
The anterior border of the tibia. It is not covered by any muscle and can be felt by touch under the skin of the anterior face of the leg.

extensor retinaculum
A fibrous ligament that crosses the anterior face of the ankle. The tendons of the muscles of the anterior face of the leg pass under this ligament to the dorsal part of the foot.

46

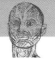

LEG. SUPERFICIAL MUSCLES

▼ POSTERIOR VIEW

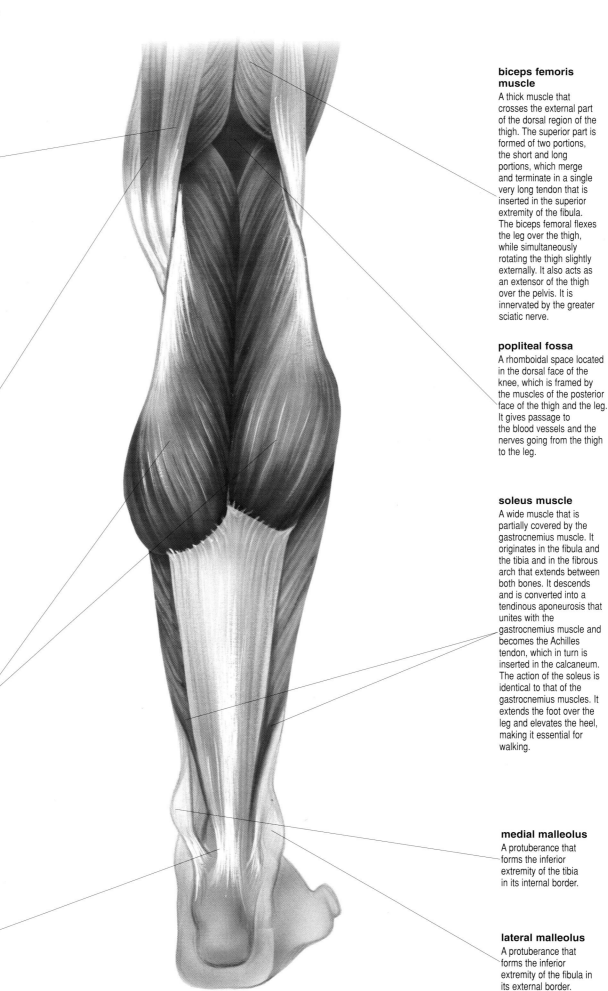

semimembranous muscle

A muscle partially covered by the semitendinosus muscle. It is called the semimembranous muscle because its superior third is composed of a wide tendinous membrane. It originates in the ischium and is inserted in the superior extremity of the tibia. Its action is similar to the semitendinosus muscle, doubling the leg on the thigh, rotating the leg inwards and extending the thigh over the pelvis.

semitendinosus muscle

A muscle with inferior and superior parts separated by a tendon. It originates in the ischium, and descends the posterior face of the thigh. After passing the internal border of the knee, it becomes anterior and is converted into the tendon known as the pes anserinus, which serves as the common insertion in the superior extremity of the tibia for two other muscles: the sartorius and the gracilis muscles. When contracted, it doubles the leg over the thigh and rotates the thigh internally. It also acts as an extensor of the thigh over the pelvis.

gastrocnemius muscle

A voluminous muscle that occupies the superficial plane of the posterior face of the leg. Superiorly it is formed by two portions, the lateral and medial heads of the gastrocnemius, which originate in the lateral and medial femoral condyles. At the height of the middle third of the leg they unite to form a single muscle that terminates in a tendinous aponeurosis which is united with the tendon of the soleus muscle to form the Achilles tendon which is inserted in the calcaneum. When contracted, these muscles extend the foot over the leg. When the heel is on the ground, they lift it while simultaneously doubling the leg over the thigh. All these actions make them essential for walking.

Achilles tendon

A tendon that serves as the common insertion of the gastrocnemius and soleus muscles. It is inserted in the posterior tuberosity of the calcaneum on the posterior part of the ankle. The Achilles is a powerful tendon that can be seen under the skin of the posterior face of the ankle.

biceps femoris muscle

A thick muscle that crosses the external part of the dorsal region of the thigh. The superior part is formed of two portions, the short and long portions, which merge and terminate in a single very long tendon that is inserted in the superior extremity of the fibula. The biceps femoral flexes the leg over the thigh, while simultaneously rotating the thigh slightly externally. It also acts as an extensor of the thigh over the pelvis. It is innervated by the greater sciatic nerve.

popliteal fossa

A rhomboidal space located in the dorsal face of the knee, which is framed by the muscles of the posterior face of the thigh and the leg. It gives passage to the blood vessels and the nerves going from the thigh to the leg.

soleus muscle

A wide muscle that is partially covered by the gastrocnemius muscle. It originates in the fibula and the tibia and in the fibrous arch that extends between both bones. It descends and is converted into a tendinous aponeurosis that unites with the gastrocnemius muscle and becomes the Achilles tendon, which in turn is inserted in the calcaneum. The action of the soleus is identical to that of the gastrocnemius muscles. It extends the foot over the leg and elevates the heel, making it essential for walking.

medial malleolus

A protuberance that forms the inferior extremity of the tibia in its internal border.

lateral malleolus

A protuberance that forms the inferior extremity of the fibula in its external border.

THE LEG. SUPERFICIAL MUSCLES

▼ EXTERNAL VIEW

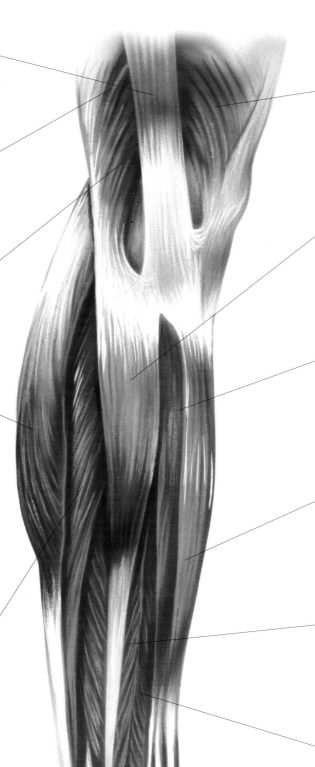

iliotibial tract
A fibrous membrane that crosses the thigh laterally and superficially and is formed by the prolongation of the membrane that covers the thigh called the fascia lata.

biceps femoris muscle
A thick muscle that crosses the external part of the dorsal region of the thigh. The superior part is formed of two portions, the short and long portions, which merge and terminate in a single very long tendon that is inserted in the superior extremity of the fibula. The biceps femoral flexes the leg over the thigh, while simultaneously rotating the thigh slightly externally. It also acts as an extensor of the thigh over the pelvis.

short portion of the biceps femoral
The short portion of the two that forms the superior part of the biceps femoris muscle. It originates in the internal border of the femur in the linea aspera.

gastrocnemius
A voluminous muscle that occupies the superficial plane of the posterior face of the leg. Superiorly it is formed by two portions, the external gemellus and the internal gemellus, which originate in the external and internal femoral condyles. At the height of the median third of the leg they unite to form a single muscle that terminates in a tendinous aponeurosis which is united with the tendon of the soleus muscle to form the Achilles tendon which is inserted in the calcaneum. When contracted, these muscles extend the foot over the leg. When the heel is on the ground, they lift it while simultaneously doubling the leg over the thigh. All these actions make them essential for walking.

soleus muscle
A wide muscle that is partially covered by the gemellus muscles and owes its name to its shape. It originates in the head, posterior face and external border of the fibula, the oblique line of the posterior face of the tibia and in the fibrous arch that extends between both bones. It descends and is converted into a tendinous aponeurosis that unites with the gemellus muscle and becomes the Achilles tendon, the common insertion of both muscles, which in turn is inserted in the calcaneum. The action of the soleus is identical to that of the gemellus muscles. It extends the foot over the leg and elevates the heel, making it essential for walking.

Achilles tendon
The common insertion of the gastrocnemius and soleus muscles. It is inserted in the tuberosity of the calcaneum in the posterior face of the ankle.

lateral malleolus
A protuberance that forms the inferior extremity of the fibula in its external border.

fibular retinaculum
A long ligament that extends from the lateral malleolus of the fibula to the external face of the calcaneum. The tendons of the long and short peroneal muscles pass under this ligament.

quadriceps femoris muscle
A thick muscle that occupies the anterior face of the thigh. It is formed of four fascicles: the vastus lateralis muscle, vastus medialis muscle, the rectus femoris muscle and the vastus intermedius muscle, which is in a deeper plane. These fascicles finish in a wide common tendinous aponeurosis that is inserted in the patella and then descends as the patellar tendon, that terminates in the anterior tuberosity of the tibia. Its main action is to extend the leg over the thigh, although it also acts to double the thigh over the pelvis.

peroneus longus muscle
A thin muscle that occupies the lateral border of the leg. It originates in the fibula and the tibia and in its inferior part becomes a tendon that passes the lateral malleolus behind to reach the sole of the foot which it crosses obliquely to be inserted in the first metatarsal. Its action is to extend the foot over the leg and to rotate the foot outwards.

extensor digitorum longus muscle
A flat muscle that shares a common origin with the anterior tibial muscle and follows a parallel trajectory until reaching the back of the foot, where it divides into four tendons that go to each of the four last toes, where they are inserted in the second and third phalanges. Its action is to extend the last four toes over the dorsal face of the foot, while simultaneously doubling the foot over the leg and turning it outwards.

peroneus brevis muscle
A muscle located below the peroneus longus muscle. It extends from the external face of the fibula to the lateral malleolus of the ankle, which it crosses posteriorly as a tendon and reaches the external area of the foot to be inserted in the fifth metatarsal. It is a separating or abductor muscle of the foot, while simultaneously rotating the foot externally.

anterior tibial muscle
A voluminous muscle that crosses the anterior surface of the leg to reach the internal border of the foot. It originates in the superior extremity of the tibia descends and converges to become a powerful tendon that passes below the extensor retinaculum and is inserted in the first metatarsal and the first cuneiform bone. When contracted, it flexes the foot over the leg, carries the foot towards the median line and rotates the foot inwards.

peroneus tertius muscle
A small, flat muscle that originates in the inferior half of the fibula. It descends to form a tendon that passes below the flexor retinaculum of the tarsus, and crosses the external border of the foot to be inserted in the fifth metatarsal. It is a flexor muscle of the foot, while simultaneously rotating and separating the foot externally.

extensor retinaculum
A fibrous ligament that crosses the anterior face of the ankle. Its internal part is formed of an inferior branch and a superior branch which further divides into deep and superficial branches. The tendons of the muscles of the anterior face of the leg pass under this ligament to the dorsal part of the foot and are stabilized by it.

THE LEG. SUPERFICIAL MUSCLES

▼ INTERNAL VIEW

semitendinosus muscle
A muscle with inferior and superior parts. It originates in the ischium, and descends the posterior face of the thigh. After passing the internal border of the knee, it becomes anterior and is converted into the tendon known as the pes anserinus, which serves as the common insertion in the superior extremity of the tibia for two other muscles: the sartorius and the gracilis muscles. When contracted, it doubles the leg over the thigh and rotates the thigh internally. It also acts as an extensor of the thigh over the pelvis.

patella
A flat, rounded bone that occupies the anterior face of the knee joint.

pes anserinus
A thick tendon that is inserted in the internal part of the superior extremity of the tibia and originates in the union of the tendons of three muscles: the sartorius, semitendinosus and the gracilis muscles. Its name means 'goose's foot', due to its shape.

anterior tibial muscle
A voluminous muscle that crosses the anterior face of the leg to reach the internal border of the foot. It originates in the superior extremity of the tibia. It descends and converges to become a powerful tendon that passes below the extensor retinaculum and is inserted in the first metatarsal and the first cuneiform bone. When contracted, it doubles the foot over the leg, carries the foot towards the median line and rotates it inwards.

tibial crest
The anterior border of the tibia. It is not covered by any muscle but is located immediately under the skin of the anterior face of the leg.

extensor retinaculum
A fibrous ligament that crosses the anterior face of the ankle. Its internal part is formed of an inferior branch and a superior branch that further divides into deep and superficial branches. The tendons of the muscles of the anterior face of the leg pass under this ligament to the dorsal part of the foot and are stabilized by it.

semimembranous muscle
A muscle partially covered by the semitendinosus muscle. It is called the semimembranous muscle because its superior third is composed of a wide tendinous membrane. It originates in the ischium and is inserted in the superior extremity of the tibia. Its action is similar to the semitendinosus muscle, doubling the leg over the thigh, rotating the thigh inwards and extending it over the pelvis.

gracilis muscle
A long, thin muscle that originates in the pubic bone and follows the internal border of the thigh to reach the superior part of the tibia, where it is inserted by a tendon that is common to two other muscles, the semitendinosus and the sartorius. The tendon is known as the pes anserinus. The gracilis muscle is a flexor of the leg over the thigh and an approximator of the thigh.

flexor digitorum longus
A muscle that originates in the posterior face of the tibia and descends as a tendon to pass behind the medial malleolus and cross the plant of the foot, where it branches into four portions which terminate in the distal phalanges of the four last toes, which they flex when contracted.

flexor hallucis longus
A muscle that follows a path parallel to the common flexor of the fingers, although it originates in the fibula. It passes behind the medial malleolus and it reaches the sole of the foot as a tendon that is inserted in the second phalange of the big toe. Its action is to flex the big toe.

deltoid ligament
The articulation of the tibia with the tarsus is reinforced in its internal face by a powerful ligament whose superficial layer has a triangular shape which gives it its name. It extends from the medial malleolus of the tibia to the calcaneum, scaphoid and talus.

flexor retinaculum
A ligament that extends from the medial malleolus of the tibia to the internal face of the calcaneum. The tendons of the flexor muscles of the posterior face of the leg pass under the ligament and are stabilized by it.

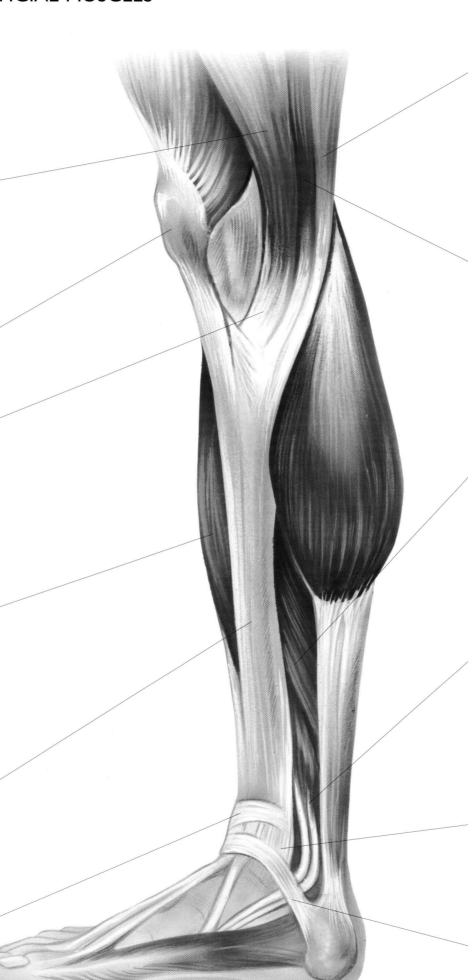

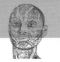

FOOT. SUPERFICIAL MUSCLES

▼ DORSAL VIEW

lateral malleolus
A protuberance formed by the inferior extremity of the fibula in its lateral border.

extensor digitorum brevis
A flat muscle that originates in the calcaneus and crosses the dorsal area of the foot obliquely. It divides into four tendons which go to the first, second, third and fourth toes. In the first toe, the tendon is inserted in the first phalanx, whereas in the other three it is united to the tendons of the common extensor muscle of the toes. Its action is to extend the four first toes over the back of the foot, collaborating with the extensor digitorum longus muscle.

tendon of the anterior peroneal muscle
A tendon whose muscular mass is located in the anterior face of the leg. It crosses the external border of the foot and is inserted in the fifth metatarsal bone. It is a flexor muscle of the foot, while simultaneously rotating and separating the foot externally.

tendons of the extensor digitorum longus muscle
The four tendons of this muscle, located in the anterior face of the leg, reach the dorsal part of the foot and go to the second and third phalanges of each of the four last toes. They act to extend the lateral four toes over the dorsal part of the foot, while simultaneously flexing the foot over the leg and moving it outwards.

tendon of the anterior tibial muscle
A tendon that comes from the anterior face of the leg, passes below the extensor retinaculum and is inserted in the first metatarsal and the first cuneiform bone. When contracted, it flexes the foot on the leg, it carries the foot towards the median line in adduction or approximation and rotates the foot inwards.

medial malleolus
A protuberance formed by the inferior extremity of the tibia in its medial border.

extensor retinaculum
A fibrous ligament that crosses the anterior surface of the ankle. It consists of inferior and superior parts. The tendons of the muscles of the anterior face of the leg pass under this ligament to the dorsal part of the foot.

tendon of the extensor hallucis longus muscle
A tendon whose muscular mass is in the anterior surface of the leg. It crosses the internal border of the dorsal part of the foot and is inserted in the first and second phalanges of the big toe. It is an extensor muscle of the big toe over the foot, and also flexes the foot over the leg and turns the foot inwards.

dorsal interosseal muscles
Four muscles in the deep plane of the plantar region, which can be visualized from the dorsal face. They are located in the intermetatarsal spaces and go to the first phalanges of the second, third and fourth toes. They act to flex the first phalanges and to extend the other two phalanges of these toes.

FOOT. SUPERFICIAL MUSCLES

▼ PLANTAR VIEW

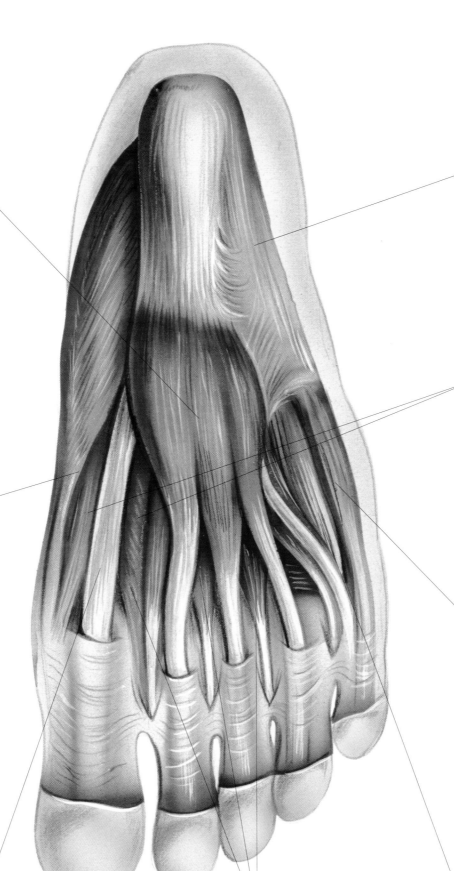

flexor digitorum brevis muscle
A muscle located in the centre of the plantar aspect of the foot. It originates in the calcaneum and divides into four fleshy bodies which become four tendons that are inserted in the second phalanges of the four last toes by thin extensions. Its action is to flex the first and second phalanges of the four last toes over the sole of the foot.

abductor hallucis
A muscle that occupies the medial border of the sole of the foot and extends from the calcaneum to the base of the first phalange of the big toe, where it is inserted by means of a tendon that is united with the tendon of the flexor hallucis longus muscle. It flexes the big toe over the sole of the foot while simultaneously separating the big and second toes.

tendon of the flexor hallucis longus
A tendon that comes from the deep plane of the posterior surface of the leg. It originates in the fibula, passes behind the medial malleolus and below the calcaneum, and is inserted in the second phalanx of the big toe. Its action is to extend the foot and to flex the phalanges of the big toe.

plantar aponeurosis
A thick, triangular membrane that covers the plantar musculature immediately below the skin, from the posterior part of the calcaneum to the base of the five toes. It emits fibrous prolongations which act as sheaths for the tendons of the flexor muscles.

flexor hallucis brevis muscle
A muscle that originates in the tarsus and divides into two bodies: one is united to the tendon of the abductor hallucis and the other to the tendon of the abductor hallucis muscle, located in the deep plane of the sole of the foot. Its action is to flex the big toe over the sole of the foot.

abductor digiti minimi
A muscle located in the lateral border of the sole of the foot, which extends from the calcaneum to the first phalange of the small toe and the fifth metatarsal. When contracted it separates the fifth toe outwards, in a movement of abduction.

flexor digiti minimi brevis muscle
A muscle that follows a path parallel to the one of the separator of the fifth toe. It extends from the base of the fifth metatarsal to the first phalange of the small toe. It collaborates with the flexor digitorum brevis muscle in the flexion of the fifth toe.

lumbrical muscles
Small cylindrical muscles that terminate in the first phalanges of each of the toes. Their action is to double the first phalange of the four last toes and to extend the other two phalanges.

51

THE SKELETON

▼ ANTERIOR GENERAL VIEW

cranium
Set of 8 flat bones
(1 frontal, 2 parietal,
2 temporal, 1 occipital,
1 sphenoid and 1 ethmoid
bone), whose articulation
comprises the cranial cavity,
which houses the brain.

mandible
A horseshoe-shaped bone, also called the
jawbone, located in the inferior part of the
face. Its articulation with the cranial
bones allows the action of chewing.

skeleton of the face
Set of bones that constitute the
skeleton of the face (1 vomer,
2 maxillae, 2 nasal, 2 palatine,
2 zygomatic, 2 lacrimal and
2 inferior nasal conchae).

1st rib
2nd rib
3rd rib
4th rib
5th rib
6th rib
7th rib
8th rib
9th rib
10th rib
11th rib
12th rib

ribs
Flat, curved bones that
surround the thoracic
cavity laterally from the
edges of the sternum to
the dorsal vertebral
column, forming the rib
cage. Eight ribs are fixed
and the other four are
joined to each other by
ligaments or have one
unattached end.

clavicles
Two long, flat bones,
located between the
sternum and the scapula
that serve as the fixation
point of the upper limbs
with the thorax.

sternum
A flat bone located in the central
anterior area of the thoracic
cavity, in which the ribs that
surround the cavity are
inserted laterally.

52

ilium
A shovel-shaped part
of the hip bone which
articulates posteriorly
with the sacrum
forming the lateral wall
of the pelvic cavity.

pubis
Part of the hip bone
that closes the
anterior part of the
pelvic cavity forming a
midline cartilaginous
joint called the
pubic symphysis.

hip bone
The bone that
composes the
skeleton of
the pelvis.
It consists
of three parts:
the ilium,
ischium and
pubis.

ischium
Part of the hip bone that
serves as the lateral
anterior union between
the pubis and the ilium.
The joint of the ischium
and the ilium forms an
articulation which
is the insertion point
of the femur.

femur
A long, thick bone that forms
the skeleton of the thigh. In
its superior part it angles
inwards to unite with the
pelvis in the hip joint.

patella
A flat, triangular bone
located in front of the
knee joint which serves as
the insertion point for
many muscles of the
thigh and the leg.

tarsus
A set of seven bones
arranged in two rows
(calcaneus, talus,
cuboid, scaphoid and
three cuneiform bones),
that constitutes the
skeleton of the
heel of the foot.

metatarsus
A set of five
long bones that
comprises the
plantar vault and
extend from the
second row of the
tarsal bones to
the phalanges of
the toes.

tibia
A long bone that forms the
internal part of the skeleton of
the leg. In its superior part it
joins the femur to form the
knee joint, and the inferior part
unites with the tarsus and the
fibula, forming the ankle joint.

fibula
A long, thin bone that forms
the external part of the
skeleton of the leg. It
articulates above and
below with the tibia.

phalanges
A set of bones that
forms the bony
skeleton of the
toes. Each toe has
three phalanges,
except the first
which has only two.

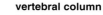

THE SKELETON

▼ POSTERIOR GENERAL VIEW

scapula
or **shoulder bone**
A flat bone located in the posterior surface of the thorax, which acts as the union between the thorax and the upper limbs.

humerus
A long bone that forms the skeleton of the arm. The upper end articulates with the scapula and the distal end with the ulna and radius.

radius
The long lateral bone of the forearm. Its upper articulation is with the humerus and the ulna in the elbow joint, and its distal articulation with the ulna and the carpal bones in the wrist joint.

ulna
A long bone that forms the medial skeleton of the forearm. It plays an important role in the rotatory movements of the forearm and hand.

carpus
A set of eight small bones (hamate, navicular, trapezium, pisiform, trapezoid, lunate, triquetrum, and capitate bones), distributed in two rows of four in the form of a cube. They articulate with the ulna and radius in the wrist joint, and with the metacarpal bones of the hand.

metacarpus
A set of five long bones that extend radially across the hand from the carpus to the phalanges of the fingers.

**phalanges
of the fingers**
A set of bones that forms the skeleton of the fingers. Each of the fingers contains three phalanges, except for the thumb, which has only two.

vertebral column
A set of 24 bones called vertebrae that articulate with one another. It is divided into three parts: cervical (7 vertebrae), thoracic (12 vertebrae) and inferior or lumbar (5 vertebrae).

sacrum
A triangular bone that forms the base of the vertebral column. Its superior articulation is with the vertebral column and the lateral articulation with the iliac bone and it thus acts as an important point of articulation which allows the inclination and extension of the thorax forwards and backwards.

coccyx
A small, terminal appendix that is located at the distal end of the sacrum and consists of a series of very small, almost atrophic vertebral vestiges.

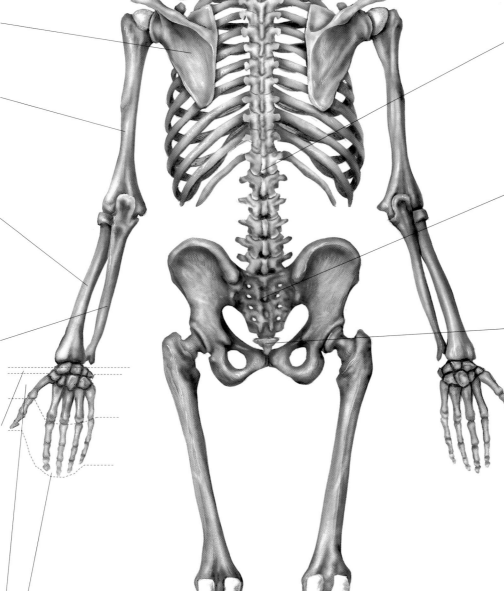

53

THE SKELETON

▶ LATERAL GENERAL VIEW

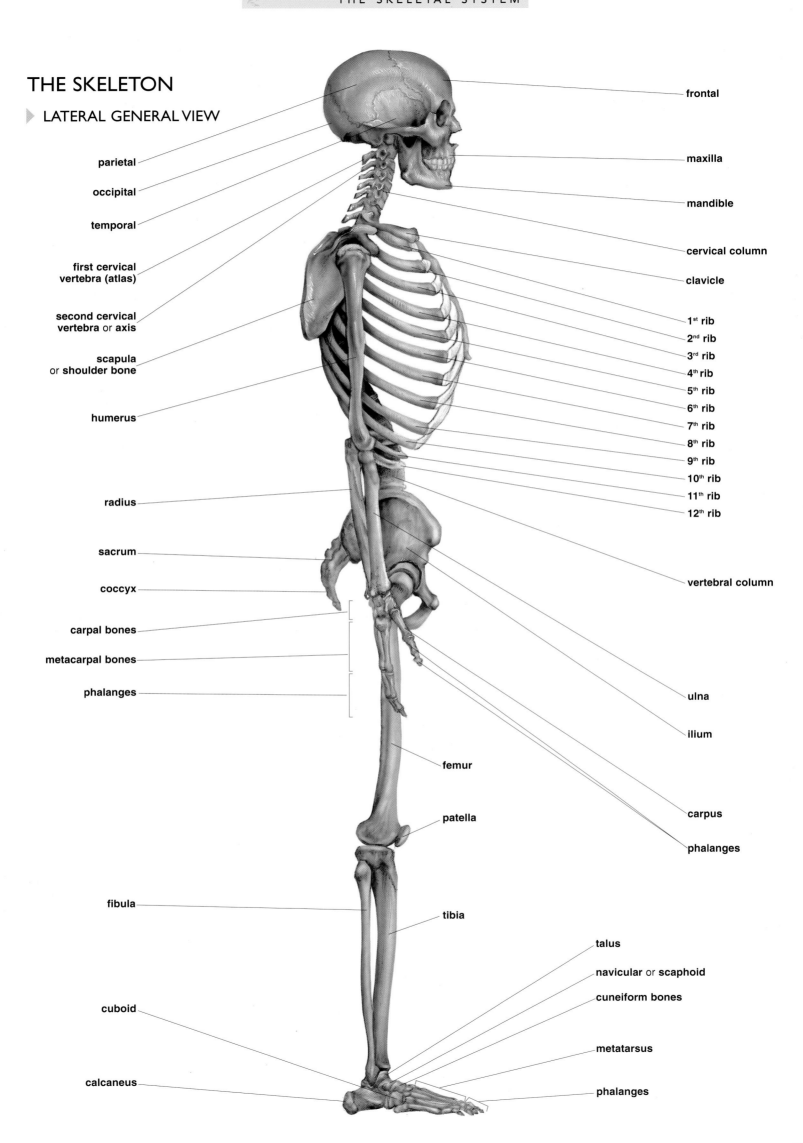

parietal

occipital

temporal

first cervical
vertebra (atlas)

second cervical
vertebra or axis

scapula
or shoulder bone

humerus

radius

sacrum

coccyx

carpal bones

metacarpal bones

phalanges

fibula

cuboid

calcaneus

frontal

maxilla

mandible

cervical column

clavicle

1st rib
2nd rib
3rd rib
4th rib
5th rib
6th rib
7th rib
8th rib
9th rib
10th rib
11th rib
12th rib

vertebral column

ulna

ilium

carpus

phalanges

femur

patella

tibia

talus

navicular or scaphoid

cuneiform bones

metatarsus

phalanges

54

THE STRUCTURE OF A LONG BONE

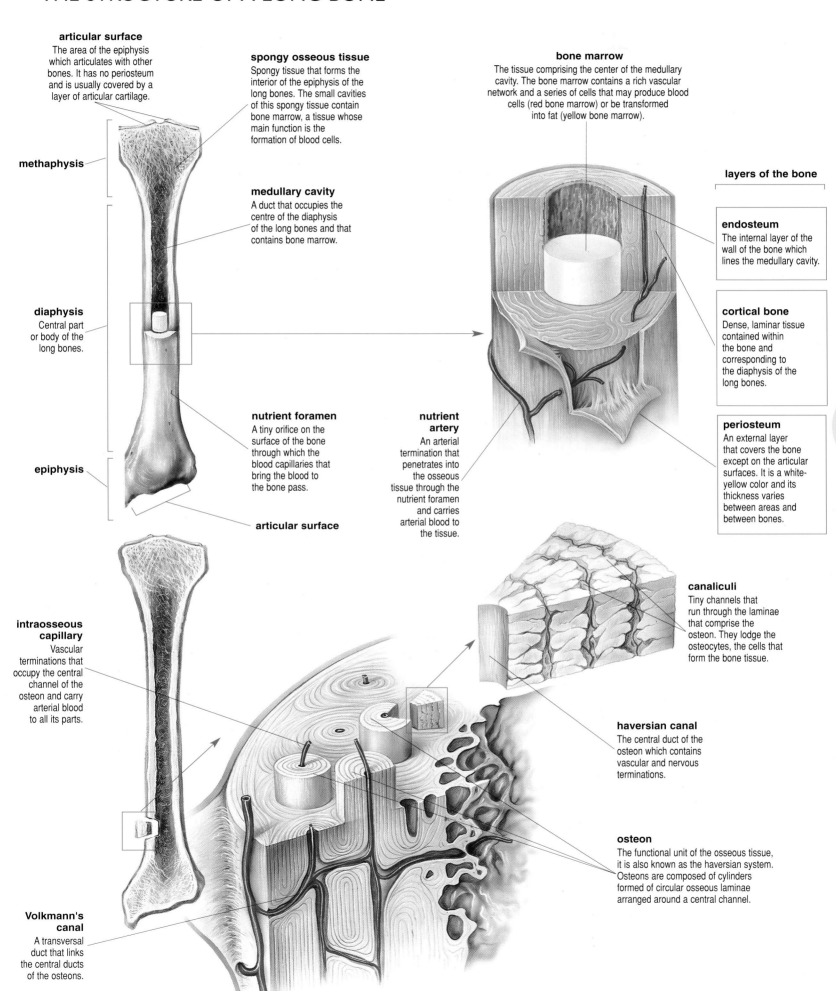

articular surface
The area of the epiphysis which articulates with other bones. It has no periosteum and is usually covered by a layer of articular cartilage.

methaphysis

diaphysis
Central part or body of the long bones.

epiphysis

spongy osseous tissue
Spongy tissue that forms the interior of the epiphysis of the long bones. The small cavities of this spongy tissue contain bone marrow, a tissue whose main function is the formation of blood cells.

medullary cavity
A duct that occupies the centre of the diaphysis of the long bones and that contains bone marrow.

nutrient foramen
A tiny orifice on the surface of the bone through which the blood capillaries that bring the blood to the bone pass.

articular surface

nutrient artery
An arterial termination that penetrates into the osseous tissue through the nutrient foramen and carries arterial blood to the tissue.

bone marrow
The tissue comprising the center of the medullary cavity. The bone marrow contains a rich vascular network and a series of cells that may produce blood cells (red bone marrow) or be transformed into fat (yellow bone marrow).

layers of the bone

endosteum
The internal layer of the wall of the bone which lines the medullary cavity.

cortical bone
Dense, laminar tissue contained within the bone and corresponding to the diaphysis of the long bones.

periosteum
An external layer that covers the bone except on the articular surfaces. It is a white-yellow color and its thickness varies between areas and between bones.

55

intraosseous capillary
Vascular terminations that occupy the central channel of the osteon and carry arterial blood to all its parts.

Volkmann's canal
A transversal duct that links the central ducts of the osteons.

canaliculi
Tiny channels that run through the laminae that comprise the osteon. They lodge the osteocytes, the cells that form the bone tissue.

haversian canal
The central duct of the osteon which contains vascular and nervous terminations.

osteon
The functional unit of the osseous tissue, it is also known as the haversian system. Osteons are composed of cylinders formed of circular osseous laminae arranged around a central channel.

THE SKULL

▼ FRONTAL VIEW

frontal bone
A large bone that forms the anterior part of the cranium and lodges, in its posterior concave face, the frontal lobes of the brain.

sphenoid bone
One of the bones that form the cranial base. In its anterior part it forms part of the wall of the orbit.

orbits
Two cavities located in the superior part of the facial skeleton which lodge the eyeballs. They are limited by the frontal bone, the sphenoid bone, the zygomatic bones, the maxillae and the lacrimal bones.

orbital fissure
An irregular cleft between the greater and lesser wings of the sphenoid bone, through which the nerves and blood vessels of the eye pass.

superciliary arch
The arches which form the superior borders of the orbits and are the bony support of the eyebrows.

zygomatic bone
One of the bones that forms the facial skeleton. It constitutes the bony support of the cheeks. Its superior edges form the floor and the external face of the orbit.

nasal septum
The osteocartilaginous plate that divides the nasal fossae. It is formed in its posterior part by the vomer bone.

maxillae
Two symmetrical bones that limit the cavity of the nasal fossae and are united in their inferior part. They also form part of the floor of the orbit and are the centre of the facial skeleton. In their inferior face they lodge the upper teeth.

mandibular angle
The angle that forms at each side of the cranium where the rami and body of the mandible meet.

teeth
Extremely hard structures arranged in two rows, with the superior row being lodged in the maxilla and the inferior row in the mandible.

mandible
The only movable bone of the head, the mandible serves as the inferior part of the face. It is articulated with the temporal bone by a joint that allows the action of chewing. The mandible has two sections: the perpendicular rami and the horizontal body.

THE SKULL

▼ LATERAL VIEW

frontosphenoidal suture
The line formed where the frontal bone meets the ala of the sphenoid bone.

external acoustic meatus
A bony canal that forms the opening in the external temporal bone which connects the cavity of the middle ear with the exterior.

coronal suture
An articulation that unites the posterior edge of the frontal bone with the anterior edges of the parietal bones.

parietal bone
Two symmetrical bones located on both sides of the cranium and united by the saggital suture.

temporoparietal suture
A fixed articulation that unites the squama of the temporal bone with the parietal bone.

temporal bone
A complex bone that contributes structurally to the cranial vault. It contains the organs of hearing and is composed of five parts: the tympanic, petrous and mastoid parts, the styloid process and the squama.

lamboid suture
The lamboid suture articulates the posterior edge of the parietal bone with the occipital bone.

occipital bone
A single, concave bone forming the posteroinferior part of the cranium. It lodges the occipital lobes of the brain and the cerebellum.

alae of the sphenoid bone
Prolongations of the sphenoid bone that form part of the temporal fossa.

nasal bones
Two flat bones, articulated by their internal faces, which form the bony support of the base of the nose.

mastoid process
The inferior protuberance of the temporal bone, which contains some irregular cavities called the mastoid cells. The mastoid process plays an important role in hearing and serves as the insertion point for many neck muscles.

glenoid cavity
The deep fossa located at the base of the temporal bone which articulates with the mandibular condyle to form the temporomandibular joint.

anterior nasal spine
The anterior prolongation of the maxillae which forms a tip and is located in the superior part of the intermaxillary suture.

condylar process of the mandible
A bony elevation of the ramus of the mandible which articulates with the glenoid cavity of the temporal bone, forming the temporomandibular joint.

zygomatic arch
A bony arch which originates in the zygomatic bone and extends laterally backwards, where it is united with the temporal bone.

coronoid process
A bony elevation located in the anterior part of the superior border of the rami of the mandible where the temporal muscle is inserted, allowing the mandible to move.

sigmoid notch
A wide notch that extends from the coronoid process to the mandibular condyle and allows the passage of vessels and nerves.

temporal fossa
A bony depression located in the lateral aspect of the cranium and formed by the ala of the sphenoid bone and the concha of the temporal bone. A large part of the temporal bone is inserted in the fossa.

styloid process
A long, thin prolongation of the inferior face of the temporal bone which serves as the insertion point for ligaments and muscles.

57

CRANIAL VAULT

▼ EXTERNAL VIEW   ▼ INTERNAL VIEW

lamboid suture
The lamboid suture articulates (joins) the posterior edge of the parietal bone with the occipital bone.

occipital bone
A single, concave bone forming the posteroinferior part of the cranium. It encloses the occipital lobes of the brain and the cerebellum.

grooves for vascular branches
Traces formed in the bone by the different blood vessels that surround the brain.

occipital fossa
The internal concavity of the occipital bone which encloses the superior part of the occipital lobe of the brain.

parietal fossae
The internal concavities of the parietal bones which enclose the parietal lobes of the brain.

coronal suture
An articulation that unites the posterior edge of the frontal bone with the anterior edges of the parietal bones.

frontal bone
A large bone that forms the anterior part of the cranium andencloses, in its posterior concave face, the frontal lobes of the brain.

saggital suture
A line of articulation that crosses the cranial vault from the frontal bone to the occipital bone, uniting the parietal bones.

parietal bone
Two symmetrical bones located on both sides of the cranium and united by the saggital suture.

longitudinal channel
A deep sulcus that serves as a prolongation of the frontal crest. It encloses the superior longitudinal sinus, an important branch of the venous system of the superior region of the cranium.

frontal crest
A bony elevation located in the central internal face of the frontal bone. It contains the falx cerebri, a membranous partition that separates the two cerebral hemispheres in this area.

frontal fossa
Internal concavity of the frontal bone in its superior part which encloses the frontal lobes of the brain.

THE BASE OF THE CRANIUM

▼ EXTERNAL VIEW

▼ INTERNAL VIEW

condyles of the occipital bone
Elevations located at both sides of the foramen magnum which articulate with the atlas.

occipital bone
A single bone forming the inferior posterior part of the cranial vault, which curves to form a concave internal surface.

temporal bone
A complex bone that contributes structurally to the cranial vault. It contains the organs of hearing and is composed of five parts: the tympanic, petrous and mastoid parts, the styloid process and the squama.

external acoustic meatus
A bony canal that forms the opening in the external temporal bone which connects the cavity of the middle ear with the exterior.

mastoid process
The inferior protuberance of the temporal bone, which contains cavities called mastoid cells. The mastoid process plays an important role in hearing.

internal auditory meatus
An orifice that opens in the internal face of the petrous bone and allows the passage of the auditory and facial nerves.

basilar part of occipital bone
An inclined channel that ends at the foramen magnum and houses the medulla oblongata.

cerebellar fossa
The depression of the interior of the occipital bone posterior to the foramen magnum which houses the cerebellum.

sella turcica
A bony structure of the sphenoid bone which partly surrounds the pituitary gland and is also known as the pituitary fossa.

foramen magnum
An oval orifice in the occipital bone which connects the cranial cavity with the spine. The medulla oblongata merges with the spinal cord at the foramen magnum.

teeth
The 16 upper teeth are inserted in the alveolar cavities of the maxilla.

sphenoid bone
One of the bones forming the cranial base. It emits prolongations called the alas of the sphenoid that comprise part of the temporal fossa.

glenoid cavity
The deep fossa located at the base of the temporal bone which articulates with the mandibular condyle to form the temporomandibular joint.

cribiform lamina
Part of the ethmoid bone that connects with the cranial cavity through tiny orifices through which branches of the olfactory nerve pass.

optic foramen
An orifice located in the internal face of the sphenoid bone which allows the ophthalmic nerve and artery to reach the orbit.

lesser alae of the sphenoid bone
Two lateral prolongations of the sphenoid bone that form the posterior wall of the orbit.

huesos maxilares superiores
Dos huesos que delimitan las fosas nasales y se unen por su parte inferior formando la bóveda palatina o cielo de la boca.

frontal crest
A bony elevation located in the central internal face of the frontal bone. It contains the falx cerebri, a membranous partition that separates the two cerebral hemispheres in this area.

frontal bone
A large bone that forms the anterior part of the cranium and encloses the frontal lobes of the brain in its posterior concave face.

59

THE VERTEBRAL COLUMN

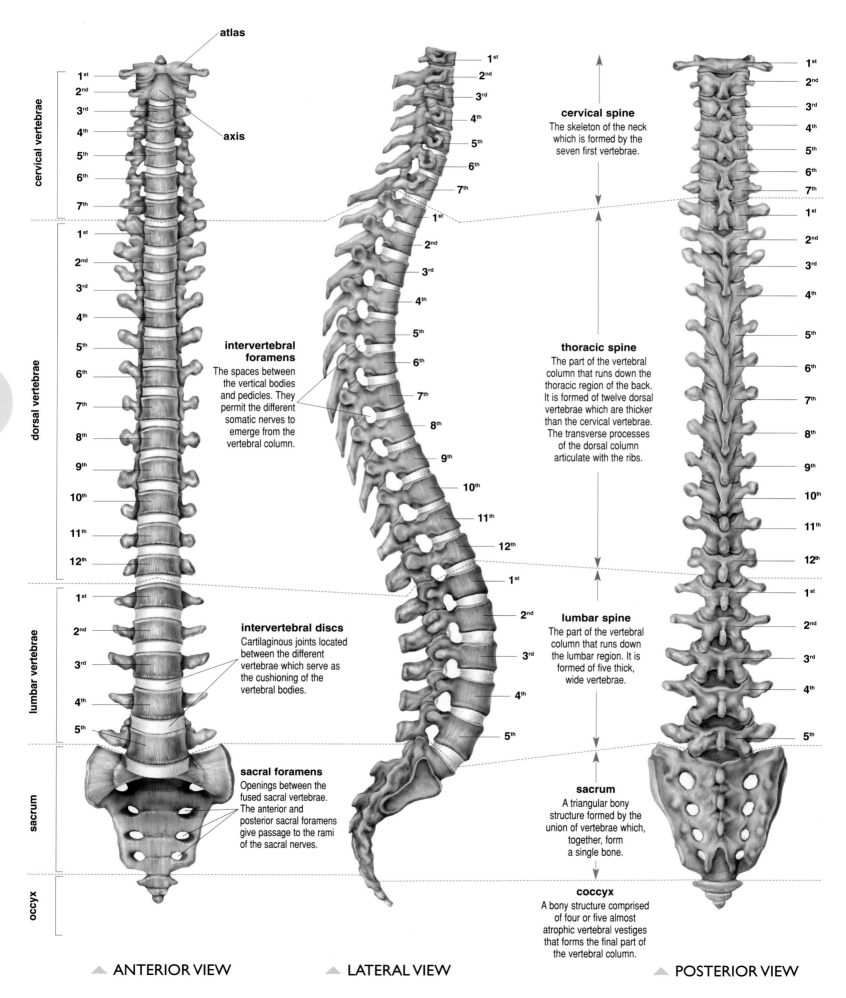

atlas

axis

cervical vertebrae
1st
2nd
3rd
4th
5th
6th
7th

dorsal vertebrae
1st
2nd
3rd
4th
5th
6th
7th
8th
9th
10th
11th
12th

lumbar vertebrae
1st
2nd
3rd
4th
5th

sacrum

occyx

intervertebral foramens
The spaces between the vertical bodies and pedicles. They permit the different somatic nerves to emerge from the vertebral column.

intervertebral discs
Cartilaginous joints located between the different vertebrae which serve as the cushioning of the vertebral bodies.

sacral foramens
Openings between the fused sacral vertebrae. The anterior and posterior sacral foramens give passage to the rami of the sacral nerves.

1st
2nd
3rd
4th
5th
6th
7th
1st
2nd
3rd
4th
5th
6th
7th
8th
9th
10th
11th
12th
1st
2nd
3rd
4th
5th

cervical spine
The skeleton of the neck which is formed by the seven first vertebrae.

thoracic spine
The part of the vertebral column that runs down the thoracic region of the back. It is formed of twelve dorsal vertebrae which are thicker than the cervical vertebrae. The transverse processes of the dorsal column articulate with the ribs.

lumbar spine
The part of the vertebral column that runs down the lumbar region. It is formed of five thick, wide vertebrae.

sacrum
A triangular bony structure formed by the union of vertebrae which, together, form a single bone.

coccyx
A bony structure comprised of four or five almost atrophic vertebral vestiges that forms the final part of the vertebral column.

1st
2nd
3rd
4th
5th
6th
7th
1st
2nd
3rd
4th
5th
6th
7th
8th
9th
10th
11th
12th
1st
2nd
3rd
4th
5th

▲ ANTERIOR VIEW   ▲ LATERAL VIEW   ▲ POSTERIOR VIEW

60

DIFFERENT TYPES OF VERTEBRAE

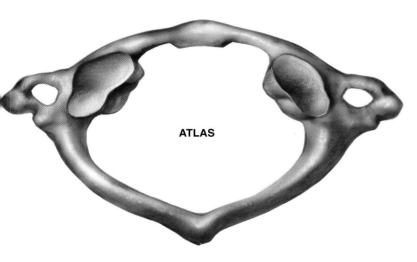

ATLAS

The first vertebra of the cervical column. Unlike the other vertebrae, it is made up of two lateral parts united by anterior and posterior arches, presenting two glenoid cavities which articulate with the occipital bone. The small face of the anterior arch articulates with the odontoid process of the axis. The transverse foramen or holes give passage to the vertebral arteries.

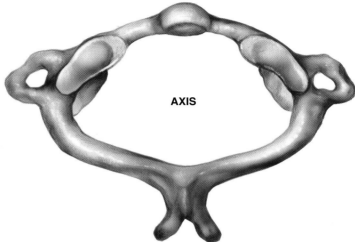

AXIS

The second cervical vertebra. It is differentiated from the other vertebrae by the fact that the vertebral body contains a prolongation known as the odontoid process, which articulates perpendicularly upwards with the atlas. The spinous process is bifurcated. Like the atlas, the axis has two lateral transverse foramen which give passage to the vertebral arteries.

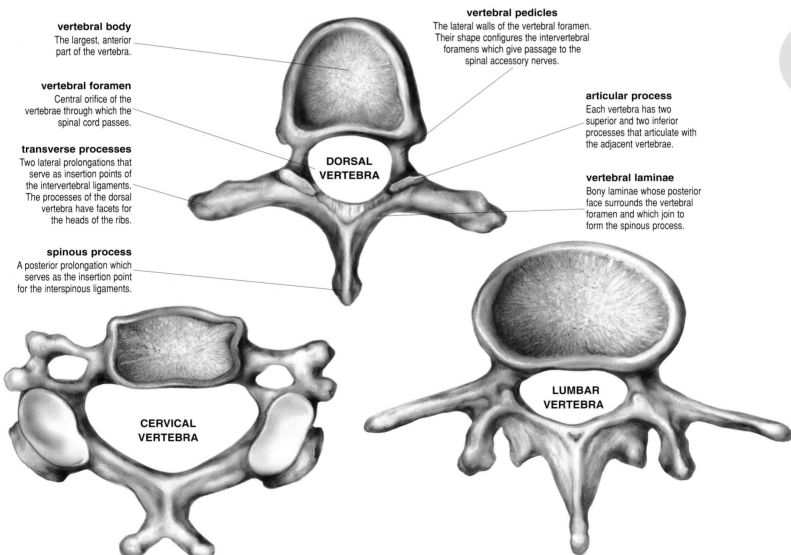

vertebral body
The largest, anterior part of the vertebra.

vertebral foramen
Central orifice of the vertebrae through which the spinal cord passes.

transverse processes
Two lateral prolongations that serve as insertion points of the intervertebral ligaments. The processes of the dorsal vertebra have facets for the heads of the ribs.

spinous process
A posterior prolongation which serves as the insertion point for the interspinous ligaments.

vertebral pedicles
The lateral walls of the vertebral foramen. Their shape configures the intervertebral foramens which give passage to the spinal accessory nerves.

articular process
Each vertebra has two superior and two inferior processes that articulate with the adjacent vertebrae.

vertebral laminae
Bony laminae whose posterior face surrounds the vertebral foramen and which join to form the spinous process.

DORSAL VERTEBRA

CERVICAL VERTEBRA

LUMBAR VERTEBRA

The differentiating characteristics of the cervical vertebrae are: the vertebral body is quadrangular, with the transversal diameter predominating; like the atlas and the axis, there are transverse holes through which the vertebral arteries pass; the spinous process is short and bifurcated and the transverse processes are implanted at the sides of the vertebral body and are short.

The characteristics of the lumbar vertebrae are: the body is very large and high; the spinous processes are well developed and descend obliquely. The lumbar vertebrae are heavily built to withstand more weight.

THE THORAX

▼ ANTERIOR VIEW

▼ POSTERIOR VIEW

manubrium
The superior part of the sternum, its superior border presents a notch called the sternal notch that can be felt under the skin. Laterally, it presents two articulate surfaces on each side, for the clavicle and the first costal cartilage.

scapula
Also known as the shoulder bone. A flat, triangular bone that joins the upper limb or extremity to the posterior part of the thorax.

clavicle
A flat, elongated bone that acts as the fixation point of the superior extremity to the sternum.

costal cartilages
Cartilaginous elements that join the ribs and the sternum.

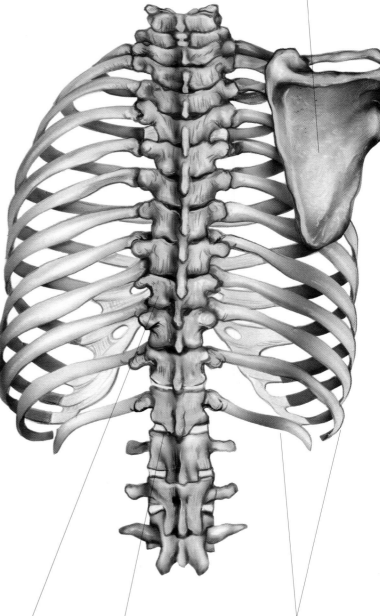

ribs
Twelve flat bones located on each side of the thorax that extend from the dorsal vertebral column to the sternum. The ribs that connect directly with the sternum are called true ribs and those which connect through a common cartilage are called false ribs.

sternum
A flat bone located in the anterior face of the thorax that serves as the anterior union of the ribs of both sides. It is divided into three parts: the manubrium, the body and the xiphoid appendix.

xiphoid appendix
Inferior end or point of the sternum which is formed of cartilaginous tissue.

body of sternum
Central segment of the sternum. It contains lateral articular faces which unite with the costal cartilages to form the sternocostal joints.

dorsal vertebral column
The bony structure formed by the twelve dorsal vertebrae. It provides posterior support to the pairs of ribs.

intervertebral discs
Cartilaginous joints located between the different vertebrae which serve to cushion the vertebral bodies.

floating ribs
The last two ribs are called floating ribs as they do not join with the sternum, leaving their anterior border free.

THE SHOULDER AND ARM

▼ ANTERIOR VIEW

▼ POSTERIOR VIEW

clavicle
A flat, elongated bone that acts as the fixation point of the superior extremity to the sternum.

greater tubercle
A large elevation located in the external zone of the neck of the humerus, which serves as an insertion point for the muscles which join the humerus with the scapula.

coracoid process
A short bony projection of the scapula. It is tipped and serves as the insertion point for the muscles and ligaments of the shoulder and arm.

lesser tubercle
A smaller elevation than the greater tubercle, located in the anterior zone of the neck of the humerus.

acromion
The projection of the scapula which constitutes the point of the shoulder. The anterior face presents a facet which articulates with the clavicle.

spine of the scapula
The posterior face of the scapula is divided by the spine of the scapula into the supraspinous and subspinous fossae.

head of the humerus
Flat, smooth surface which forms almost a third of a sphere and which articulates with the glenoid cavity of the scapula.

anatomical neck of the humerus
A constricted area just below the head of the humerus which joins the head to the body.

scapula
A flat triangular bone which, with the clavicle, forms the pectoral girdle.

glenoid cavity
Oval articular face located at the upper lateral angle of the scapula which articulates with the head of the humerus.

humerus
A long, heavy bone that forms the skeleton of the arm. It consists of the head, which is articulated with the scapula to form the shoulder joint, the body, and the lower extremity which articulates with the ulna and radius and forms the elbow joint.

medial epicondyle
A projection of the inner part of the distal extreme of the humerus, also known as the internal condyle.

olecranon fossa
A cavity located over the trochlea in its posterior face. It accommodates the extremity of the olecranon, or the superior part of the articular extremity of the ulna when in extension.

humeral condyle
A hemispheric projection located in the external part of the lower extremity of the humerus. It articulates with the head of the radius.

coronoid fossa
A cavity located over the trochlea in its anterior face which receives the coronoid process of the ulna when the elbow is flexed.

humeral trochlea
An articular surface in the form of a pulley, located in the lower extremity of the humerus, which articulates with the sigmoid cavity of the ulna.

63

THE FOREARM

▼ ANTERIOR VIEW

▼ POSTERIOR VIEW

greater sigmoid cavity
Hook-shaped articular cavity which articulates with the humeral trochlea.

coronoid process
The anterior end of the greater sigmoid cavity, which ends in a tip that articulates with the coronoid fossa of the humerus when the forearm is flexed.

radial tuberosity
A bony protuberance located below the neck of the radius that serves as the insertion for one of the tendons of the biceps muscle of the arm.

neck of the radius
A somewhat narrower part of the radius that joins the body of the bone to the head.

olecranon
Superior extreme of the greater sigmoid cavity which finishes in a tip that is articulated in the olecranon fossa of the humerus.

head of radius
The superior extremity of the radius is cylindrical. The superior face is concave and is called the glenoid cavity of the radius. The internal part of the cylinder articulates with the ulna.

head of the ulna
A thickened, hemispheric area which forms the inferior extreme of the ulna. In its external part it articulates with the radius and in the inferior part with the pyramidal bone of the carpus.

styloid process of the radius
A thick prolongation located in the inferior extremity of the radius, and which can be felt beneath the skin. It serves as an insertion point for ligaments and muscles of the wrist and forearm.

styloid process of the ulna
A cylindrical prolongation that extends sertically downwards from the inferior extremity of the ulna and serves as the insertion point for some of the ligaments of the wrist joint.

ULNA
The long bone that occupies the inner part of the forearm and plays a fundamental role in the rotation of the forearm and hand. It consists of a central body and two extremes. The superior extreme is very voluminous and forms part of the articulation of the elbow while the inferior extreme is part of the wrist joint.

RADIUS
A long bone that forms the external part of the skeleton of the forearm. It consists of a central body and two extremes. The superior extreme forms part of the elbow joint, and the larger, inferior extreme forms part of the wrist joint.

64

THE HAND

pisiform
A vertically elongated bone located in the internal extremity of the superior row of the carpus.

triquetrum
A bone in the centre part of the superior row of the carpus which is shaped like a pyramid.

lunate
A bone shaped like a half-moon and located in the centre of the superior row of the carpus.

capitate
The largest of the carpal bones, which occupies a central place in the inferior row of the carpus.

navicular
The largest and most external of the bones that form the superior row of the carpus.

carpal bones
A set of eight articulated bones arranged in two rows. They articulate with the ulna and the radius above and with the metacarpal bones below.

sesamoid
Small bones with a fibrous structure which are found in varying numbers in the joints of the hand.

trapezoid
A small bone located in the centre part of the inferior row of the carpus.

hamate
The medial bone of the four bones that form the inferior row of the carpus. It has an anterior hook-shaped projection.

trapezium
A bone located in the lateral aspect of the inferior row of the carpus.

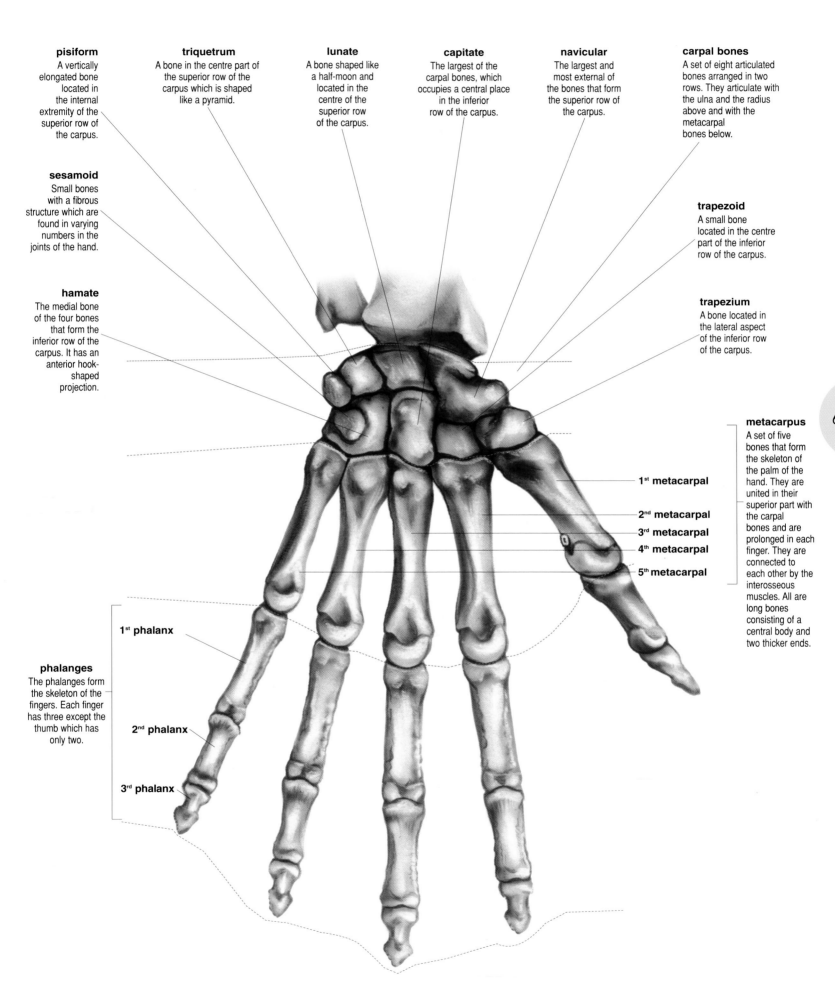

65

metacarpus
A set of five bones that form the skeleton of the palm of the hand. They are united in their superior part with the carpal bones and are prolonged in each finger. They are connected to each other by the interosseous muscles. All are long bones consisting of a central body and two thicker ends.

1st metacarpal
2nd metacarpal
3rd metacarpal
4th metacarpal
5th metacarpal

1st phalanx

phalanges
The phalanges form the skeleton of the fingers. Each finger has three except the thumb which has only two.

2nd phalanx

3rd phalanx

THE PELVIS

▼ POSTERIOR VIEW

hip bone
The three bones of the hip, the ilium, ischium and pubis, form the innominate bone. The two symmetrical innominate bones form the hip bone, also called the pelvic girdle or pelvis. The bones are united posteriorly with the sacrum and anteriorly with each other by the pubic symphysis.

ilium
The external part of the hip bone, which is shaped like a shovel. It forms the lateral wall of the pelvic cavity.

ischium
The ischium forms the inferior part of the hip bone and consists of a voluminous body and an ascending branch which is united with the descending branch of the pubis.

pubis
The internal part of the hip bone.The pubis consists of a central body, a horizontal branch that articulates with the cotyloid cavity and a descending branch. The two pubic bones are connected.

iliac crest
A bony crest that forms the superior border of the ilium and extends from the sacroiliac joint to the anterior superior iliac spine.

external iliac fossa
A wide surface located in the posterior part of the ilium which serves as an insertion point for the gluteus muscles.

sciatic spine
An elevation located below the greater sciatic notch which serves as an insertion point for muscles and ligaments.

sacrum
A triangular bony structure. A single bone formed by the union of five vertebrae. It is located at the base of the vertebral column and articulates laterally with the hip bones.

sacroiliac joint
A joint with almost no mobility which unites the articular face of the sacrum with an ear-shaped facet of the internal part of the ilium called the auricular surface.

greater sciatic notch
A large notch located in the posterior border of the ilium through which a large number of blood vessels and nerves leave the pelvis.

coccyx
A rudimentary structure which is the vestige of the tail in human beings. It is formed of four or five atrophic fused vertebrae.

obturator foramen
Also called the lesser sciatic foramen. A large orifice located below the acetabulum which is limited by the ischium and the pubis. It is covered by a fibrous lamina called the obturator membrane.

66

▼ ANTERIOR VIEW

iliac crest
A bony projection located in the external border of the ilium which can be felt through the skin of the hip.

anterior inferior iliac spine
A bony projection that appears below the iliac crest. It serves as the insertion for a muscular tendon.

interior iliac fossa
A triangular surface that serves as the insertions for the iliac muscle and corresponds to the internal part of the ilium.

pubic symphysis
A joint that articulates the two pubic bones and which closes the anterior face of the pelvic cavity.

acetabulum
Cavity located in the centre of the hip bone which forms a ball-and-socket joint with the femoral head. It is surrounded by the ilium (superior zone), the pubis (anterior inferior zone) and the ischium (posterior inferior zone).

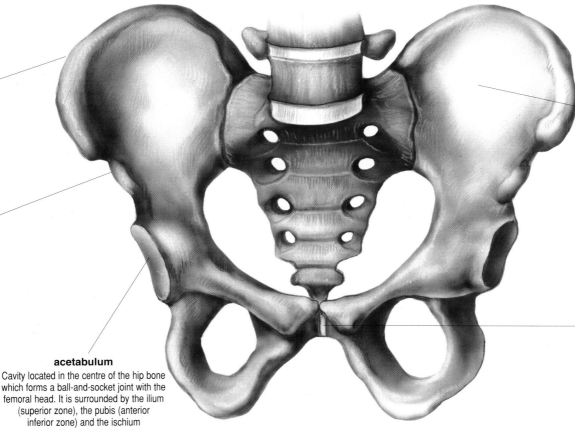

THIGH AND KNEE

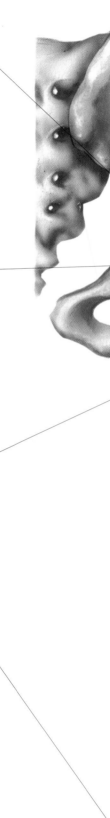

**head
of the femur**
Smooth, almost
spherical surface
that articulates with
the acetabulum of
the hip bone in a
ball-and-socket joint
to form the hip joint.

**anatomical
neck of the
femur**
A narrower area that
joins the head of the
femur to the rest of
the bone.
It is shaped like a
flattened cylinder
and serves as an
insertion point for
the ligaments and
capsule of the
hip joint.

hip joint
The joint formed
by the head of the
femur and the
acetabulum of the
hip bone.

**greater
trochanter**
A thick
eminence
located in the
posterior
external part of
the base of the
anatomical neck
of the femur
which serves as
the insertion
point for several
groups of
muscles.

**lesser
trochanter**
An elevation
located in the
posterior medial
part of the base of
the anatomical
neck of the femur
which serves as
the insertion point
for some of the
muscles that unite
the pelvis with
the femur.

FEMUR

A long bone that forms the
skeleton of the thigh. It is
the longest bone in the
human body and consists
of a central body and two
extremities. The superior
extreme forms part of the
hip joint, and the inferior
extreme forms part
of the knee joint.

**femoral
trochlea**
Articular surface in
the shape of a
pulley with a
central notch that
extends along the
inferior extreme of
the femur and
articulates with the
superior part
of the tibia.

patella
A short, flat bone
located in the anterior
area of the knee. It
presents a convex
anterior face and a
slightly concave
posterior face
containing two
articular facets that
articulate with the
femoral condyles. In
its superior part, the
tendon of the rectus
femoris muscle is
inserted and in the
inferior part the
prolongation of this
tendon, called the
patellar ligament,
is inserted.

**medial
condyle**
Tuberosity located
in the medial part
of the lower
extremity of the
femur which
articulates with the
internal glenoid
cavity of the tibia.
In its lateral zone it
presents a
tuberosity that
serves as the
insertion for the
knee ligaments.

lateral condyle
A tuberosity located
in the lateral part of
the lower extremity
of the femur which
articulates with the
lateral articular
surface of the tibia.
It presents a lateral
tuberosity to which
articular ligaments
are inserted.

67

▲ ANTERIOR VIEW

▲ POSTERIOR VIEW

THE LEG

head of the fibula
The superior part of the fibia is larger than the rest. The medial part contains an articular facet which articulates with the upper extremity of the tibia.

intercondylar tuberule
An elevated projection that separates the lateral and medial articular faces of the tibia and articulates with the femoral trochlea.

articular surfaces of the tibia
Two slightly concave articular surfaces, one lateral and the other medial, located in the superior face of the tibia, which articulate the lateral and medial condyles of the femur, respectively.

anterior tibial tuberosity
A projection located in the superior part of the anterior border of the tibia in which the patellar ligament is inserted.

styloid process of the fibula
A bony projection that extends vertically upwards from the head of the fibula. The tendon of biceps femoris inserts here.

tibial crest
The anterior border of the tibia which crosses the anterior part of the body of the bone longitudinally. It has no muscular insertions and can be felt through the skin.

FIBULA

A long bone that forms the external part of the skeleton of the leg. It has a body and two extremes, the superior and inferior, that articulate with the tibia, to form the superior and inferior tibiofibular joints. The inferior extreme also articulates with the talus.

TIBIA

A long bone that comprises the internal skeleton of the leg. It has a long central body and two extremes. The large, superior extreme forms part of the knee joint, and the smaller, inferior extreme forms part of the ankle joint.

lateral malleolus of the fibula
A bony projection located in the external part of the inferior extremity of the fibula, immediately below the skin. It is furrowed by a channel that gives passage to the tendons of the muscles of the fibula.

medial tibial malleolus
A thick projection located in the medial area of the tibia and forming part of the ankle joint. It serves as an insertion point for various ligaments.

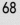

68

▲ ANTERIOR VIEW

▲ POSTERIOR VIEW

THE FOOT

▼ DORSAL VIEW

▼ PLANTAR VIEW

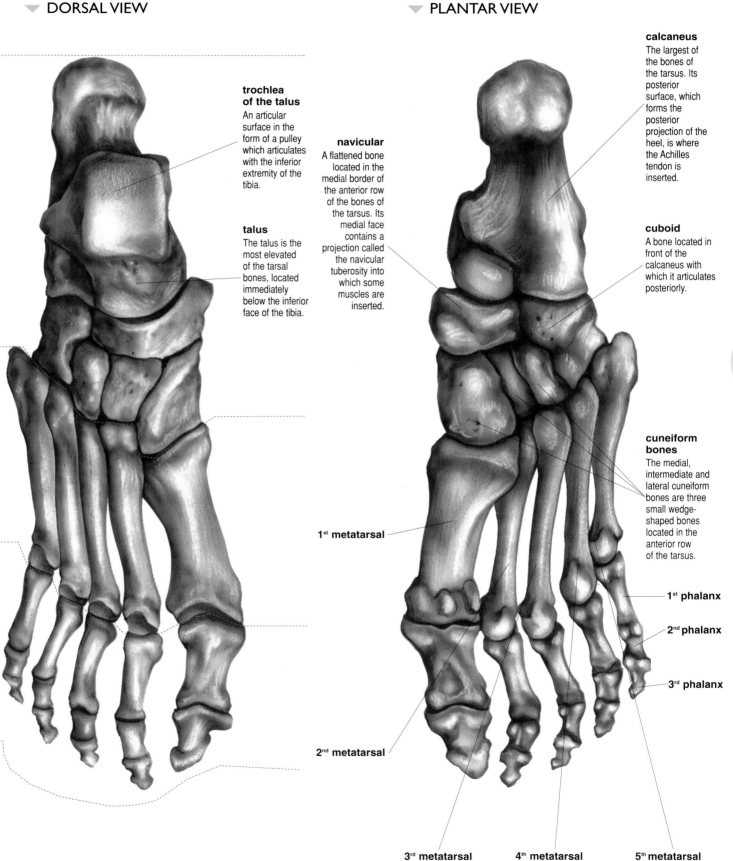

tarsus
The tarsus is a set of seven articulated short bones which is joined superiorly with the tibia and fibia and inferiorly with the metatarsal bones. The tarsus, considered in its totality, has the shape of a concave vault. Its movements are fundamental for the dynamics of the foot.

metatarsus
A set of five long bones, that are united posteriorly with the bones of the tarsus and which are prolonged in their inferior part along each toe. They consist of a central body with a triangular cross-section which is slightly curved and concave, and two heavier ends.

phalanges of the toes
The phalanges constitute the skeleton of the toes. Each toe consists of three phalanges, which are called, from top to bottom, the first, second and third phalanges, except for the thumb, which has only two. They are long bones, somewhat shorter than the phalanges of the fingers, although they have the same morphologic characteristics, with a long body and two thicker extremes.

trochlea of the talus
An articular surface in the form of a pulley which articulates with the inferior extremity of the tibia.

talus
The talus is the most elevated of the tarsal bones, located immediately below the inferior face of the tibia.

navicular
A flattened bone located in the medial border of the anterior row of the bones of the tarsus. Its medial face contains a projection called the navicular tuberosity into which some muscles are inserted.

calcaneus
The largest of the bones of the tarsus. Its posterior surface, which forms the posterior projection of the heel, is where the Achilles tendon is inserted.

cuboid
A bone located in front of the calcaneus with which it articulates posteriorly.

cuneiform bones
The medial, intermediate and lateral cuneiform bones are three small wedge-shaped bones located in the anterior row of the tarsus.

1st metatarsal

2nd metatarsal

3rd metatarsal

4th metatarsal

5th metatarsal

1st phalanx

2nd phalanx

3rd phalanx

69

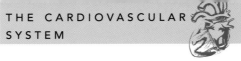

ARERIAL SYSTEM

▼ ANTERIOR GENERAL VIEW

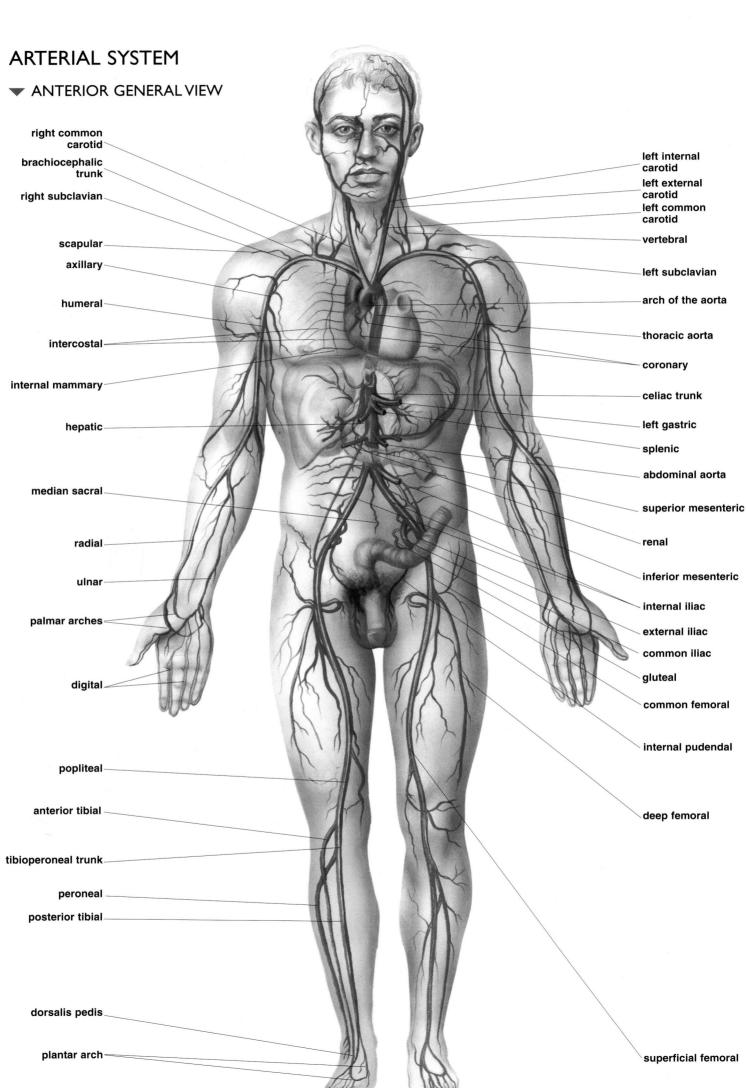

right common carotid

brachiocephalic trunk

right subclavian

scapular

axillary

humeral

intercostal

internal mammary

hepatic

median sacral

radial

ulnar

palmar arches

digital

popliteal

anterior tibial

tibioperoneal trunk

peroneal

posterior tibial

dorsalis pedis

plantar arch

left internal carotid

left external carotid

left common carotid

vertebral

left subclavian

arch of the aorta

thoracic aorta

coronary

celiac trunk

left gastric

splenic

abdominal aorta

superior mesenteric

renal

inferior mesenteric

internal iliac

external iliac

common iliac

gluteal

common femoral

internal pudendal

deep femoral

superficial femoral

70

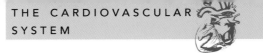

VENOUS SYSTEM

▼ ANTERIOR GENERAL VIEW

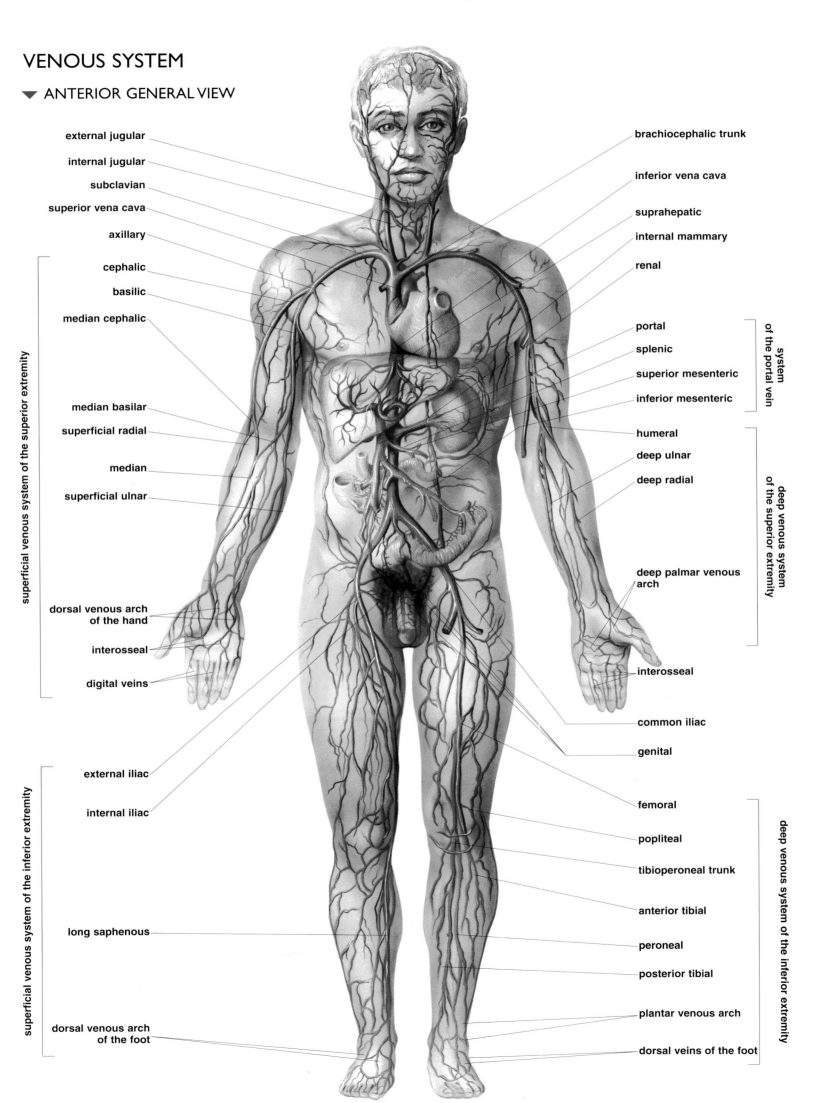

external jugular
internal jugular
subclavian
superior vena cava
axillary
cephalic
basilic
median cephalic

superficial venous system of the superior extremity

median basilar
superficial radial
median
superficial ulnar

dorsal venous arch of the hand
interosseal
digital veins

brachiocephalic trunk
inferior vena cava
suprahepatic
internal mammary
renal
portal
splenic
superior mesenteric
inferior mesenteric

system of the portal vein

humeral
deep ulnar
deep radial

deep venous system of the superior extremity

deep palmar venous arch
interosseal
common iliac
genital

superficial venous system of the inferior extremity

external iliac
internal iliac
long saphenous
dorsal venous arch of the foot

femoral
popliteal
tibioperoneal trunk
anterior tibial
peroneal
posterior tibial
plantar venous arch
dorsal veins of the foot

deep venous system of the inferior extremity

71

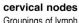
LYMPHATIC SYSTEM

▼ ANTERIOR GENERAL VIEW

LYMPHATIC SYSTEM

The lymphatic system is an accessory route for the transport of fluids and the substances they contain, especially proteins, coming from the tissues of the body. It acts as a complementary system of the arterial and venous system and has its own network that transports the lymphatic fluid or lymph, to the blood.

cervical nodes
Groupings of lymph nodes that filter lymphatic fluid from the head. They are located in the lateral area of the neck, in the submaxillary region, the area of the nape of the neck, the parotid region and other cervical regions.

axillary nodes
A large group of nodes located under the skin of the axilla. They filter the lymph from the superior extremity before the lymph reaches the venous blood.

subclavian veins
The right and left subclavian veins channel the blood from the axillary veins of the arms. They pass below the clavicles to unite with the jugular veins and then the superior vena cava through the brachiocephalic venous trunks. The subclavian veins receive the great lymphatic vein (right) and the thoracic lymph duct (left).

lymph nodes
Thickenings of the lymphatic vessels which are distributed throughout the network. Their function is to filter the lymph and to purify it of foreign bodies. Although they exist in all areas of the body, they are more common in certain areas such as the inguinal, axillary and cervical regions, etc.

right lymphatic duct
A lymphatic duct located in the superior right area of the thorax, which receives the lymphatic vessels of the right half of the head and thorax and right upper extremity. It joins the right subclavian vein.

thoracic lymph duct
A thick lymphatic duct that passes through the abdomen and the thorax vertically, parallel to the aorta, and joins the left subclavian vein near its union with the jugular vein. It collects the lymph coming from the inferior extremities, the intestine, the left half of the thorax, the left arm and half of the left side of the head.

cisterna chyli
A dilated saccular expansion in the lower part of the thoracic duct located posterior to the aorta into which the two lumbar lymphatic trunks and the intestinal trunk open.

inguinal ganglia
The inguinal area is especially rich in lymph nodes which filter the lymph coming from the inferior extremities.

Peyer's patch
Large aggregates of lymphoid tissue or lymph nodes found in the small intestine, which are part of the lymphatic system that helps to fight infection.

lymphatic vessels
Ducts that cover all the body, closely paralleling the venous system, that collect the lymph coming from the lymphatic capillaries.

lymphatic capillaries
Small ducts similar to the venous capillaries, which begin in the sinuses of all body tissues and collect the lymph to transport it to the larger lymphatic vessels.

72

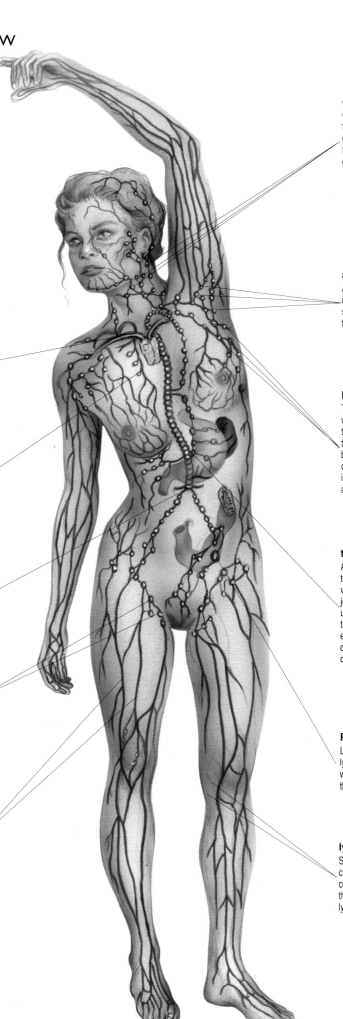

ARTERIES AND VEINS. INTERNAL STRUCTURE

ARTERIES

Blood vessels that carry the blood oxygenated in the lungs (arterial blood) to the tissues of the body. The arteries become smaller as they extend through the body until terminating in arterioles and arterial capillaries.

arterioles

Very small vessels that are the continuation of the successive ramifications of the arteries, and which carry the blood to the arterial capillaries. Their tunic media is formed by a thin muscular lamina.

capillaries

Microscopic ramifications of the arteries that carry the arterial blood to all parts of the body and facilitate the exchange of oxygenated blood and venous blood. At their extremes, they are united with the venous capillaries, which collect deoxygenated blood and transport it to the venous system.

VEINS

Blood vessels that carry the deoxygenated or venous blood, loaded with waste products, from the body tissues to the heart and lungs, where it will be oxygenated. The venous system includes the small venous capillaries, venules and medium-sized and large veins.

venules

Very small veins that join the medium and large-size veins and result from the progressive union of the different capillaries.

venous capillaries

A network of microscopic blood vessels that are the origin of the venous system. They collect the blood containing waste products from the different body tissues and transport it to the venules and larger veins.

73

tunica intima or endothelium

The tunica intima is the internal layer of the venous and arterial walls and rests on a layer of connective tissue.

tunica adventitia

The outer layer of the arteries and veins. It is formed of connective tissue and includes the nervous terminations and the blood capillaries that reach the arteries and veins.

subendothelial layer

A layer located between the tunica intima and tunica media, which is well developed in large arteries and contains many elastic fibres, giving it a striated aspect.

tunica media

The middle layer of the three that form the arterial wall. It is composed of smooth muscular fibres arranged concentrically, and is especially abundant in the medium-sized arteries. In the larger arteries, this layer contains a large amount of elastic fibres that allow the artery to contract and expand to adapt to changes in the blood volume due to the contraction and relaxation of the heart.

tunica media

The intermediate layer of the vein wall which, unlike that of the arteries, has very few muscular fibres but a large amount of collagen fibres. Only the veins of the inferior half of the organism have a certain amount of muscular fibres that facilitate the ascent of the venous blood.

valves

Folds of the internal wall of the veins, which are distributed throughout the system. Their function is to allow the blood to pass in the direction of the heart and to prevent any reflux of venous blood.

THE HEART

▼ ANTERIOR SUPERFICIAL VIEW

**left common
carotid artery**
A large artery that originates in
the arch of the aorta and carries
the arterial blood to the left half of
the head and the neck.

**brachiocephalic
arterial trunk**
A thick, ascending
arterial branch that
originates in the arch of
the aorta. Its branches
carry oxygenated blood
to the right arm and
right half of the neck
and the head.

left subclavian artery
Superior branch of the arch of
the aorta which carries arterial
blood to the left arm.

aorta
The aorta is the largest artery in
the body. It originates in the left
ventricle and first ascends and
then curves downwards in the
arch or the aorta, and crosses
the diaphragm to arrive at the
abdomen. The aorta carries all
the oxygenated blood from
the heart and distributes it
throughout the body.

pericardium
A fibrous sac that covers
all the heart, including
the trunk of the aorta and
the other large heart
vessels (superior and
inferior vena cava,
pulmonary artery and
veins, etc.).

left pulmonary artery
A branch of the pulmonary
artery which originates
in the right ventricle. It takes
the venous blood to the left
lung, where it is oxygenated
and the carbon dioxide
eliminated.

**superior
vena cava**
A thick venous trunk that
receives the veins of the
arms and the head and
carries their venous
blood to the right atrium.

pulmonary artery
A thick trunk that originates in
the right ventricle and divides
into left and right branches
that take the venous blood to
the respective lungs.

**right pulmonary
artery**
A branch of the pulmonary
artery that originates in
the right ventricle. It carries
the deoxygenated blood to
the right lung, where it is
oxygenated and the carbon
dioxide eliminated.

left atrium
The superior cavity of
the heart, which receives
the blood oxygenated in the
lungs from the pulmonary
veins. It has relatively
thin walls.

right atrium
A cavity with thin walls which
collects the venous blood
coming from the superior and
inferior vena cava.

left coronary artery
A branch of the aorta which
descends bordering the left side
of the heart through the sulcus
between the atrium and the left
ventricle. It has branches which
go to the interventricular area
and the left side of the heart.

**atrioventricular
or coronary sulcus**
A fold or sulcus that forms
the separation between
the two atriums and two
ventricles of the heart.

great cardiac vein
A vein that occupies
the atrioventricular sulcus
collecting the venous
blood of the branches
of the left side of the body
and transporting it to
the coronary sinus.

small cardiac vein
A vein that travels through
the atrioventricular sulcus
collecting the blood from
the venous branches of
the right side of the body
and carrying it to the
coronary sinus.

right coronary artery
A branch of the aorta originating in
the anterior surface of the heart
which crosses the right side of the
heart through the atrioventricular
sulcus and carries arterial blood to
the posterior face of the heart. It
has branches that go to
the right border and posterior face
of the heart and another
interventricular branch.

**marginal branch
of the
coronary artery**
An arterial branch
originating in the right
coronary artery which
carries oxygenated
blood to all the right
side of the heart.

right ventricle
The inferior cavity of
the heart, which receives
the venous blood from
the right atrium and
sends it through
the pulmonary artery to
the lungs. It has thick
muscular walls.

**interventricular
coronary artery**
A branch of the left
coronary artery that
descends the anterior
face of the heart
in the area of
the interventricular
septum.

left ventricle
A large cavity that receives
the oxygenated blood from the
left atrium and, by means of
powerful contractions of its
thick walls, sends it through
the aorta to all the body.

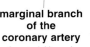

THE HEART

▼ INTERNAL VIEW

aorta
A large artery that transports all the arterial blood from the left ventricle to distribute it throughout the body.

aortic valve
A valve located in the communicating orifice between the left ventricle and the aorta. Its opening in systole (ventricular contraction) allows the oxygenated blood to reach the aorta, and its closing in diastole (ventricular relaxation) closes this circulation and prevents the blood returning from the aorta to the ventricle.

left pulmonary vein
One of the four blood vessels, two from the right lung and two from the left, which carry the oxygenated blood from the lungs to the left atrium.

left atrium
One of the two superior cavities of the heart, formed by thin walls whose superior part contains the orifices of the four pulmonary veins. These deliver the blood from the lungs to the heart. It connects with the left ventricle through the mitral valve.

superior and inferior vena cava
The superior and inferior vena cava join at the level of the right atrium in which they deposit the venous blood from all the body.

coronary arteries
The arterial system that runs through all the heart.

mitral valve
A valvular system equipped with two valves that separates the left atrium from the left ventricle. Its opening and closing permits the blood to flow from the atrium to the ventricle but not from the ventricle to the atrium.

right atrium
A cavity with thin walls located in the superior area of the heart. It receives the venous blood from all the body from the venae cava. It connects with the immediately inferior cavity, the right ventricle, through the tricuspid valve.

pericardium
The pericardium is a fluid-filled sac that surrounds the heart and the proximal part of the aorta, vena cava and the pulmonary artery. It is divided into three layers, the fibrous, visceral and parietal pericardium.

myocardium
The walls of the heart are composed mainly of cardiac muscle cells called the myocardium, which enable the heart to contract and relax. The myocardium is very thick around the ventricles and thinner around the atria. It contains the nerves which mark the rhythm of the heart movement.

tricuspid valve
A valvular system that separates the right atrium from the right ventricle. It opens to permit blood to flow from the atrium to the ventricle and contracts to prevent blood flowing from ventricle to atrium. The opening and closing of the heart valves creates a click which is the sound of the heart beats that can be heard through a stethoscope.

endocardium
The innermost layer of the wall of the heart. It is a thin layer of connective tissue made of endothelial cells which covers all the structures of the heart.

papillary muscles
Muscular columns that serve as a prolongation of the mitral and tricuspid valves and which are attached to the ventricular walls, facilitating the movement of the valve by their contractions.

interventricular septum
A thick wall of powerful muscular tissue that separates the two ventricular cavities completely and is responsible for their movements. The superior part becomes thinner and is more fibrous.

left ventricle
A cavity with thick walls that receives the oxygenated blood from the left atrium and, by means of strong contractions, expels it towards the arterial system, which carries it through the body. As the effort of the left ventricle is greater than that of the right, the muscular walls are thicker.

right ventricle
A large cavity located in the inferior part of the heart. It has thick muscular walls and its function is to store the venous blood coming from the right atrium and to send it, by means of abrupt contractions, towards the lungs, where it is oxygenated and purified.

THE ARTERIAL SYSTEM. AORTA

AORTA

The largest artery, which carries the blood flow to all parts of the human body. It originates in the right ventricle and, after ascending, forms a descending curve called the arch of the aorta, crosses the thorax as the thoracic aorta. It crosses the diaphragm, to become the abdominal aorta, which, near the pelvic cavity divides into the common iliac arteries which irrigate the inferior extremities.

right brachiocephalic trunk

A thick arterial trunk that originates in the right part of the arch of the aorta and rapidly bifurcates into an ascending branch, which carries the blood to the head (right common carotid artery), and a horizontal branch, which carries blood to the right superior extremity (subclavian artery).

left common carotid artery

Unlike the right side of the body, the left side does not posses a common brachiocephalic trunk. The left common carotid artery originates directly in the arch of the aorta and ascends through the neck to the left part of the head, bifurcating into the internal and external carotid arteries.

renal arteries

Two arteries that branch laterally and horizontally from the aorta and go to the kidneys.

hepatic artery

The hepatic artery is a branch of the celiac trunk and supplies the liver.

genital arteries

Two arteries that descend to the testicles in men (testicular arteries) or the ovaries in women (ovarian arteries).

lumbar arteries

Five arteries that branch perpendicularly from the abdominal aorta and supply the muscles and other structures of the walls of the abdominal cavity.

abdominal aorta

The name given to the section of the aorta that crosses the diaphragm and enters the abdominal cavity. The first branches go to the diaphragm and later branches include the celiac trunk, the renal arteries, the superior and inferior mesenteric arteries, etc. The abdominal aorta terminates in a bifurcation into the common iliac arteries.

right subclavian artery

The horizontal branch of the bifurcation of the brachiocephalic trunk. It originates all the arteries that irrigate the right superior extremity.

right common carotid artery

The ascending branch of the bifurcation of the brachiocephalic trunk. It branches into the internal and external right carotid arteries which irrigate the intra- and extracranial structures of the right side of the head.

left vertebral artery

The ascending branch of the left subclavian artery which ascends through the neck parallel to the cervical vertebral column and enters the skull through the foramen magna, originating the arterial network that irrigates the posterior part of the brain and cerebellum.

inferior thyroid artery

The inferior thyroid artery originates in the left subclavian artery and ascends through the neck. It has branches that go to the oesophagus, trachea, larynx and thyroid.

left subclavian artery

The left subclavian artery carries arterial blood to the left superior extremity. It originates directly in the arch of the aorta, unlike the right side of the body where a common brachiocephalic trunk supplies the blood to the head and the right superior extremity.

arch of the aorta

On leaving the left ventricle, the aorta first ascends and then immediately turns left forming an arch which descends. The branches of this region of the aorta supply all the arterial blood to the head and superior extremities.

thoracic aorta

The portion of the aorta that crosses the thoracic cavity vertically from the arch of the aorta to the diaphragm. It has branches that go to the oesophagus, the bronchi, the mediastinum and the intercostal areas.

intercostal arteries

Horizontal branches of the thoracic aorta which enter the intercostal spaces laterally. There are twelve intercostal arteries plus posterior branches to the vertebrae and anterior branches to the intercostal muscles, pleura, ribs, etc.

celiac trunk

A thick arterial trunk that originates in the front part of the abdominal aorta. It supplies arterial blood to the liver, stomach and spleen through the hepatic, gastric coronary and splenic arteries.

splenic artery

The left branch of the celiac trunk which supplies the spleen.

gastric coronary artery or stomachic

A branch of the celiac trunk that irrigates the internal area of the stomach.

superior mesenteric artery

An artery found below the origin of the celiac trunk and also in the anterior surface of the abdominal aorta. It irrigates the small intestine, a part of the pancreas and the mesentery, and the right portion of the large intestine.

inferior mesenteric artery

An artery that supplies the left part of the large intestine, from the middle of the transverse colon to the rectum, through successive ramifications (colic, sigmoid, haemorrhoidal arteries, etc.).

common iliac arteries

The common iliac arteries originate in the final bifurcation of the abdominal aorta and descend obliquely towards the inferior extremities. At the level of the sacroiliac union, they bifurcate into internal and external branches. Other branches go to some of the pelvic muscles of the abdominal cavity.

76

THE ARTERIAL SYSTEM. ABDOMEN

superior pancreatoduodenal artery
An arterial branch that originates in the superior mesenteric artery and goes to the duodenum and the left part of the pancreas.

middle colic artery
The median colic artery originates in the superior mesenteric artery and irrigates the transverse colon. It forms an arterial network which unites with the branches of the inferior mesenteric artery.

superior mesenteric artery
An artery that appears below the origin of the celiac trunk and also in the anterior face of the abdominal aorta. It irrigates the small intestine, a part of the pancreas and the mesentery, and the right portion of the large intestine.

inferior pancreatico-duodenal artery
An arterial branch of the superior mesenteric artery that irrigates the inferior border of the pancreas.

abdominal aorta
The name given to the section of the aorta that crosses the diaphragm and enters the abdominal cavity. The first branches go to the diaphragm and later branches include the celiac trunk, the renal arteries, the superior and inferior mesenteric arteries, etc. The abdominal artery terminates in a bifurcation into the common iliac arteries.

right colic artery
The right colic artery originates in the right side of the superior mesenteric artery and divides into branches which go to the ascending colon.

inferior mesenteric artery
An artery that supplies the left part of the large intestine, from the middle of the transverse colon to the rectum, through successive ramifications (colic, sigmoid, haemorrhoidal arteries, etc.),

ileocolic artery
A branch of the superior mesenteric artery which, like the right colic artery, goes to the ascending colon and also has branches to the final part of the ileum.

left colic artery
The left colic artery originates in the inferior mesenteric artery and supplies the descending colon. It has some branches that supply part of the transverse colon, uniting with branches of the superior mesenteric artery.

jejunal and ileal arteries
A series of arterial branches that go to the ileum and jejunum through a series of arches which cross the mesentery.

sigmoid arteries
The sigmoid arteries arise from the inferior mesenteric artery and supply the final part of the large intestine: the sigmoid colon, rectum and anus.

common iliac artery
The common iliac arteries originate in the bifurcation of the abdominal aorta and descend obliquely towards the inferior extremities. At the level of the sacroiliac union, they bifurcate into internal and external branches. Other branches go to some of the pelvic muscles of the abdominal cavity.

haemorrhoidal arteries
Arteries originating in the inferior mesenteric artery that go to the final part of the anus and constitute the haemorrhoidal plexus. A part of this area is irrigated by arteries coming from the internal iliac artery.

77

external iliac artery
The most external branch of the common iliac artery is divided. It crosses the pelvic cavity obliquely to reach the inguinal area and becomes the arteries of the inferior extremity. It has branches to the ureter and abdomen and a branch that ascends by the anterior wall of the abdomen called the epigastric artery.

internal iliac artery
The common iliac artery bifurcates into two branches, the internal and external iliac arteries. The internal iliac, also called the hypogastric artery, goes to the viscera of the pelvic cavity such as the bladder and uterus (intrapelvic branches) and to the external genitals and the internal part of the thigh (extrapelvic branches).

THE ARTERIAL SYSTEM. HEAD AND NECK

superficial temporal artery
One of the branches of the external carotid artery at the level of the mandibular joint. It ascends through the temporal area, has branches that supply the face, the mandibular joint, the auricular region and the orbital area, then bifurcates into frontal and parietal branches.

parietal artery
The posterior branch of the bifurcation of the superficial temporal artery. It has numerous branches which go to the parietal area of the skull.

frontal artery
The anterior branch of the bifurcation of the superficial temporal artery. It goes to the forehead where it has numerous branches.

internal maxillary artery
The internal maxillary artery originates in the terminal bifurcation of the external carotid, passes under the zygomatic arch, enters the skull through the sphenopalatine foramen and goes to the nasal septum and conchae. It has numerous branches that supply the tympanum, the temporal fossa, the dental and buccal area, the palate, the masseter muscle and the pharynx. In the skull it also has meningeal branches.

posterior auricular artery
An artery that originates from the posterior aspect of the internal carotid artery and has branches supplying the parotid gland. It terminates in a bifurcation with branches going to the mastoid and auricular regions.

occipital artery
The occipital artery originates from the posterointernal aspect of the external carotid artery and goes posteriorly to the occipital area.

vertebral artery
A branch of the subclavian artery which supplies the musculature of the cervical vertebral area. It ascends through the neck and enters the cranium through the foramen magna. It has branches going to the meninges, medulla oblongata and cerebellum.

facial artery
A branch of the external carotid artery that borders the mandible and goes to the face passing close to the commissure of the lips and terminating in the internal angle of the eye. It has submental branches and other facial branches which go to the masseter muscle, the superior and inferior lips and the area of the ala of the nose.

internal carotid artery
The postero-medial tranch of the common carotid artery. It ascends and enters the cranium through the carotid foramen. The internal carotid has multiple branches that irrigate the brain, the eyeball (ophthalmic artery) and other intracranial structures.

lingual artery
The anterior branch of the external carotid artery, which passes below the mandible and goes to irrigate the muscles of the tongue.

external carotid artery
The external carotid artery originates at the bifurcation of the common carotid artery and goes to the area of the mandibular joint, where it generates two terminal branches that go to the maxilla, the temporal area and the auricular area. It also has collateral branches that go to the thyroid, larynx, tongue, etc.

subclavian artery
The external branch of the bifurcation of the brachiocephalic trunk. It goes to the arm and supplies all the arterial circulation of the superior extremity.

right brachiocephalic trunk
A thick arterial trunk that originates in the highest part of the arch of the aorta and immediately bifurcates into the common carotid artery, which supplies the head, and the subclavian artery, which supplies the superior extremity.

common carotid artery
A branch of the brachiocephalic trunk that ascends following the lateral border of the neck and carries the blood to one side of the head. It branches into the external and internal carotid arteries.

superior thyroid artery
Shortly after the external carotid artery arises from the common carotid, it gives rise to the superior thyroid artery, which descends and supplies the thyroid. Its branches go to the larynx, the sternocleidomastoid muscle and the muscles of the inferior area of the hyoid bone.

THE ARTERIAL SYSTEM. CRANIAL BASE

**anterior cerebral
artery**

The anterior cerebral artery
is a branch of the internal
carotid. It runs above
the optic nerve to the corpus
callosum and is joined by the
anterior communicating artery
shortly after its origin. It
has branches that pass to
the anterior part of the internal
capsule and basal nuclei.

**middle cerebral
artery**

The middle cerebral artery
originates in the internal
carotid and goes laterally
to the external face of the
brain. It supplies a part of
the frontal lobe, the temporal
lobe and the parietal lobe of
the brain, both superficially
and deeply.

**posterior cerebral
artery**

The posterior cerebral artery
originates in the anterior
bifurcation of the basilar
artery and, after passing the
cerebral peduncle, goes
laterally and posteriorly to
the inferior surface of the
occipital and temporal lobes,
with deep branches to
the interior of these areas.

basilar artery

The basilar artery
originates in the union
of the two vertebral
arteries and goes
anteriorly to bifurcate
into the two posterior
cerebral arteries.

vertebral artery

The artery that carries blood to the posterior
part of the intracranial structures. It
originates in the subclavian artery and, after
ascending through the neck, it enters in the
skull through the foramen magna and goes
to the central area where the two vertebral
arteries are united to form the basilar artery,
which, in turn branches into the median and
posterior cerebellar arteries and the anterior
spinal artery.

anterior spinal artery

The anterior spinal artery is one of
the major arteries to the spinal cord and
is formed from branches of the vertebral
arteries which unite in the median fissure
of the spinal cord. It runs the length
of the cord.

**posterior inferior
cerebellar artery**

A branch of the vertebral artery
that follows a winding passage
through the inferior face of the
cerebellum, supplies this area.

circle of Willis

A polygonal figure formed by
the union of different arteries
of the base of the cranium. It
contains the optical chiasm
and the hypophysial stem
which unites the hypophysis
with the brain. The sides of
the polygon are formed by
the anterior cerebral arteries,
united by the anterior
communicating artery,
the posterior cerebral arteries
and the posterior
communicating arteries.

**internal carotid
artery**

An artery that provides
a large part of the cerebral
circulation. It enters the
skull from the neck through
the carotid foramen.
Its main branches are
the ophthalmic artery,
the anterior cerebral artery
and the middle cerebral
artery.

**posterior
comunicating
artery**

An arterial branch of
the internal carotid artery
which terminates in the
posterior cerebral artery,
communicating the two
arterial systems that
irrigate the brain,
the internal carotid
and vertebral arteries.

**superior
cerebellar artery**

It originates from the
basilar artery and goes
to the superior surface
of the cerebellum.

**anterior inferior
cerebellar artery**

This artery originates
in the basilar artery,
close to the union of
the basilar and vertebral
arteries, and goes to
the anteroinferior area
of the cerebellum.

THE ARTERIAL SYSTEM. SHOULDER AND ARM

anterior circumflex humeral artery
A thin arterial branch that originates from the axillary artery and passes in front of the humerus. It supplies the shoulder joint, the deltoid muscle, the biceps and other muscles of the area.

brachial artery
The brachial artery is a continuation of the axillary artery, which goes from the area of the axilla to the elbow, where it divides into a lateral or radial branch and a medial or cubital branch. It also has branches that go to the muscles of the arm, nutrient branches to the humerus and several other collateral branches.

radial collateral artery
A large artery that originates in the brachial artery. It passes behind the humerus and descends the posterior face of the arm to its external area, passing the elbow and uniting with the anterior radial recurrent artery. It has various branches that go to the triceps muscle.

radial recurrent artery
An artery that branches from the radial artery shortly after its beginning, and follows a retrograde or ascending path to unite with the deep humeral artery. It supplies the epicondyle muscles of the external part of the elbow and forearm.

radial artery
An artery that originates in the bifurcation of the brachial artery in the flexure of the elbow. It follows the lateral border of the forearm to the carpus. It has branches that go to the muscles of the anterior part of the arm and the carpal area.

axillary artery
When the subclavian artery passes the clavicle it becomes the axillary artery which crosses the axilla to the arm. It has mammary, thoracic and chest and scapular branches that remain in the region of the thorax and the shoulder, and circumflex branches which go to the arm.

posterior circumflex humeral artery
A branch of the axillary artery which passes behind the humerus, carrying blood to the triceps, some shoulder muscles and the deltoid muscles.

superior ulnar collateral artery
An artery that originates in the brachial artery and descends along the medial aspect of the arm to reach the elbow, where it is united with the anterior ulnar recurrent artery. It has small branches that go to the internal part or vastus medialis of the triceps.

inferior ulnar collateral artery
A thin artery that branches from the brachial artery and goes to the elbow, where it divides into anterior and posterior branches that are united with the anterior and posterior recurrent ulnar arteries, respectively. It irrigates the muscles of the internal area of the elbow and forearm or the epitrochlear muscles.

anterior recurrent ulnar artery
An artery that branches from the ulnar artery shortly after its beginning, and follows a retrograde or ascending path to unite with the anterior branch of the inferior ulnar collateral artery. There is also a posterior ulnar recurrent artery that follows a parallel path along the upper surface of the elbow.

ulnar artery
The medial branch of the bifurcation of the brachial artery. It passes along the medial border of the forearm to the palmar area. It supplies the posterior area of the forearm and reaches the interosseal region of the hand.

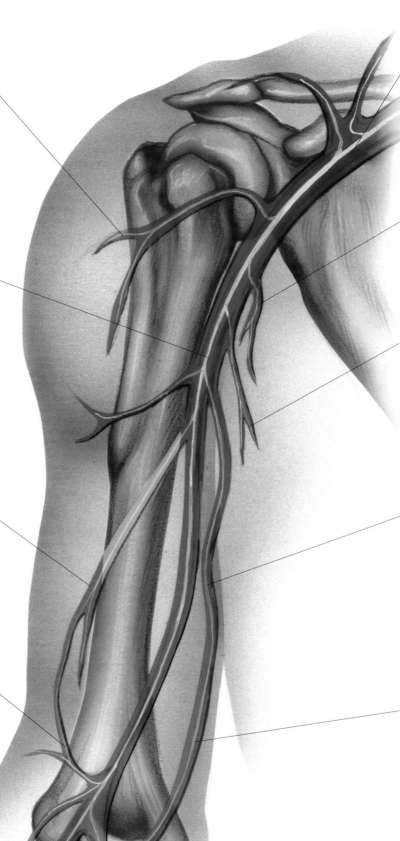

80

THE ARTERIAL SYSTEM. FOREARM AND HAND

radial recurrent artery
An artery that branches from the radial artery shortly after its beginning, and follows a retrograde or ascending path to unite with the deep humeral artery. It supplies the epicondyle muscles of the external part of the elbow and forearm.

radial artery
An artery that originates in the bifurcation of the humeral artery in the flexure of the elbow. It follows the lateral border of the forearm to the carpus. It has branches which go to the muscles of the external part of the forearm and the carpal area.

palmar branch of the radial artery
A branch of the radial artery that originates near to the wrist and goes to the palm of the hand and is united with the termination of the ulnar artery to form the superficial palmar arch.

artery of the thumb
A branch of the radial artery which goes to the thumb whose posterior surface it crosses.

common digital palmar arteries
Arteries that branch from the superficial palmar arch and follow a parallel path to the metacarpal bones, reaching the beginning of the fingers, where they are transformed into the proper palmar digital arteries.

proper palmar digital arteries
Arteries that originate in the common digital palmar arteries. There are two for each finger, and they run along the external and internal borders of the fingers.

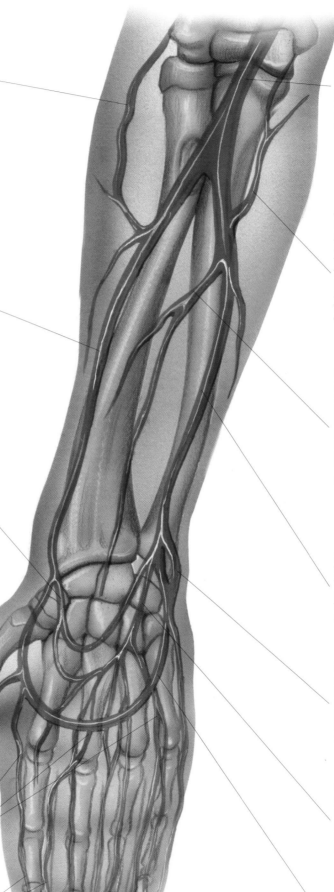

brachial artery
An artery proper to the arm which is a continuation of the axillary artery, going from the axilla to the elbow, where it divides into an external branch, the radial artery and an internal branch, the ulnar artery. It has branches to the muscles of the arm, nutritional branches to the humerus and several other collateral branches.

anterior ulnar recurrent artery
An artery that branches from the ulnar artery shortly after its beginning, and follows a retrograde or ascending path to unite with the anterior branch of the inferior ulnar collateral artery. There is also a posterior ulnar recurrent artery that follows a parallel path along the dorsal surface of the elbow.

interosseal artery
A branch of the ulnar artery which goes to the space between the ulna and the radius. It bifurcates into an anterior branch, which remains in the anterior face of the forearm, and a posterior branch, which crosses the ligament uniting both bones and passes to the dorsal surface. The two branches carry blood to the majority of the muscles of the forearm.

ulnar artery
The internal branch of the bifurcation of the humeral artery. It passes along the medial border of the forearm to the palmar area, with branches that supply the muscles of these areas.

palmar branch of ulnar artery
A branch of the ulnar artery which goes to the palm of the hand where it is united with the termination of the radial artery, giving rise to the deep palmar arch. It has small branches which go to the muscles of the hypothenar eminence.

superficial palmar arch
Formed by the union of the palmar branch of the radial artery, a branch of the radial artery, with the termination of the ulnar artery. The arch gives rise to the digital arteries which carry blood to the fingers.

deep palmar arch
The result of the union of the palmar ulnar artery, a branch of the ulnar artery, with the termination of the radial artery. Its branches are the interosseal arteries that unite with the digital arteries.

81

THE ARTERIAL SYSTEM. THIGH

inguinal ligament
A fibrous ligament that extends from the anterosuperior iliac spine to the pubis. The arteries, veins and nerves of the inferior extremity pass under the arch to the thigh.

common femoral artery
A continuation of the external iliac artery, which begins in the inguinal area and goes to the thigh, where it bifurcates into a superficial femoral artery and a deep branch. It emits branches to the genital area called the pudendal branches and others to the walls of the abdomen.

external or **anterior circumflex**
A branch of the deep femoral artery that extends outwards and irrigates the muscles of this area and the hip joint.

deep femoral artery
A branch of the common femoral artery that goes between the muscles of the thigh to become posterior. It emits ramifications to the head of the femur and the quadriceps, adductor and flexor muscles.

popliteal artery
A continuation of the femoral artery that begins at the top of the popliteal fossa, which it crosses vertically. It sends branches to the knee joint and the gastrocnemius muscle and divides into the anterior tibial artery and the tibioperoneal trunk.

external iliac artery
The external branch of the two into which the common iliac artery divides. It crosses the pelvic cavity obliquely to reach the inguinal area and has branches to the ureter and abdomen and a branch that ascends the anterior wall of the abdomen called the epigastric artery.

internal iliac artery
The internal iliac artery, also called the hypogastric artery, goes to the organs of the pelvic cavity such as the bladder and uterus (intrapelvic branches) and to the external genitals and the internal part of the thigh (extrapelvic branches).

internal or **posterior circumflex artery**
It originates from the back face of the deep femoral artery and passes behind the humerus going to the inferior part of the gluteal region.

superficial femoral artery
From its origin in the bifurcation of the common femoral artery, the superficial femoral crosses the medial aspect of the thigh and when it reaches the popliteal fossa, becoming the popliteal artery. Its branches go to the quadriceps muscle.

genicular artery
An artery that originates from the superficial femoral artery, and descends the internal border of the thigh to bifurcate into a superficial or saphenous branch and another deep or articular branch.

THE ARTERIAL SYSTEM. LEG AND FOOT

popliteal artery
A continuation of the femoral artery that begins at the height of the popliteal fossa, which it crosses vertically. It sends branches to the knee joint and the gastrocnemius muscle and divides into the anterior tibial artery and the tibiofibular trunk.

genicular artery
An artery that originates in the superficial femoral artery, and descends the internal border of the thigh to bifurcate into a superficial or saphenous branch and another deep or articular branch.

anterior tibial recurrent artery
A branch of the anterior tibial artery which irrigates the area of the knee.

tibioperoneal trunk
A short section of artery which results from the bifurcation of the popliteal artery and goes to the posterior area of the leg, dividing into the posterior tibial artery and peroneal artery.

posterior tibial artery
A branch of the internal bifurcation of the medial tibioperoneal trunk. It descends the posteromedial side of the leg, emitting branches that go to the muscles of the area and the tibia. It crosses the ankle joint and gives rise to the plantar arteries of the foot.

anterior tibial artery
A branch of the popliteal artery which becomes anterior after crossing the interosseal space located between the tibia and the fibula. It continues along the external part of the leg, crosses the ankle, and goes to the dorsum of the foot. It has branches that go to the peroneal muscles, the areas of the internal and lateral malleoli, and a recurrent or retrograde branch that goes to the knee.

peroneal artery
It originates in the tibioperoneal trunk and goes to the posterolateral area of the leg where it supplies the muscles of the area and the fibula and reaches the heel of the foot.

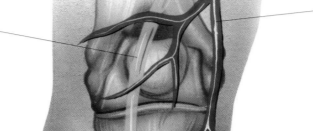

dorsalis pedis artery
A continuation of the anterior tibial artery which begins at the dorsal area of the foot. It supplies the tarsus and metatarsus and emits branches that are united with the plantar arteries, forming the plantar arch.

internal malleolar artery
A branch of the anterior tibial artery which irrigates the area of the medial malleolus.

internal and external plantar arteries
Terminal branches of the posterior tibial artery that cross the internal and external borders of the foot and are united to form the plantar arch.

external malleolar artery
A branch of the anterior tibial artery which irrigates the area of the lateral malleolus.

plantar arch
An arch that crosses the sole of the foot, formed by the union of the plantar arteries of the posterior tibial artery and the terminal branches of the dorsalis pedis artery. The arch gives rise to the interosseal arteries and those that irrigate the toes.

interosseal arteries or metatarsals
Arteries that originate in the plantar arch and continue in the interosseal spaces of the four last metatarsals, emitting branches that reach the toes.

83

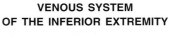

THE VENOUS SYSTEM. FOOT AND LEG. SUPERFICIAL VEINS

**subcutaneous veins of the
anterior surface of the knee**
A dense venous network that
ascends the leg just below the skin and carries
the venous blood of this area
to the great saphenous vein.

VENOUS SYSTEM
OF THE INFERIOR EXTREMITY

The superior and inferior extremities are
equipped with twin venous systems, one deep
and the other superficial. The deep venous system
is a parallel system to the arterial system, with
identical names and trajectory, although there
are two veins for each artery. For these reasons
it is not considered necessary to illustrate it.
The superficial venous system, on the contrary,
has a different trajectory and nomenclature and
runs up the leg in more superficial areas although
it terminates in the deep venous system.

**opening of the short saphenous
vein in the popliteal vein**
When it reaches the popliteal fossa in
the posterior part of the knee, the small
saphenous vein terminates in the popliteal
vein, part of the deep venous system
of the inferior extremity.

small saphenous vein
A vein that originates in the external part
of the dorsal venous arch of the foot and
after passing behind the lateral malleolus
of the ankle, ascends the posterior area of
the leg and reaches the thigh, where it
unites with the popliteal vein of the deep
venous system. It also has a branch that
terminates in the great saphenous vein.

**communication between the
external and long saphenous veins**
When it passes the knee posteriorly, the short
saphenous vein terminates in the popliteal vein
of the deep venous system, but it also has a
communicating branch that unites it with the
long saphenous vein.

**subcutaneous veins of
the anterior face of the leg**
A dense venous network that
crosses the knee and the leg just
below the skin and carries the
venous blood of this area to
the long saphenous vein.

dorsal venous arch of the foot
A venous network located in the superficial
area of the back of the foot, formed by the
confluence of the digital veins and some
plantar veins. It ascends internally
to the great saphenous vein and
externally to the external saphenous.

long saphenous vein
A vein that originates in the medial
part of the dorsal venous arch of the foot
and, after passing in front of the medial
malleolus of the ankle, ascends the
leg, collecting the venous blood of the
subcutaneous venous network of the
anterior and internal part of the leg.
After passing the knee it reaches the
thigh, crossing superficially in its
anterointernal sur face to terminate in
the femoral vein.

veins of the toes
Small veins that originate in
the extremities of the toes, basically
on the dorsal surface, and which carry
the venous blood of this area
to the dorsal arch of the foot.

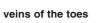

84

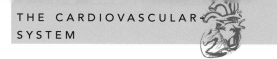

THE VENOUS SYSTEM. THIGH. SUPERFICIAL VEINS

**VENOUS SYSTEM
OF THE INFERIOR EXTREMITY**

The superior and inferior extremities are equipped with twin venous systems, one deep and the other superficial. The deep venous system is a parallel system to the arterial system, with identical names and trajectory, although there are two veins for each artery. For these reasons it is not considered necessary to illustrate it. The superficial venous system, on the contrary, has a different trajectory and nomenclature and runs up the thigh in more superficial areas, although it terminates in the deep venous system.

circumflex iliac vein
A vein that follows a parallel path to the artery of the same name and collects the venous blood from the superficial area of the lateral walls of the abdomen. It terminates in the femoral vein.

external iliac vein
A thick vein that is a continuation of the femoral vein. It receives the venous blood from the inferior extremity and carries it to the inferior vena cava, where the internal iliac vein also terminates.

femoral vein
The superficial and deep venous systems of the leg and thigh converge in the femoral vein, which ascends the thigh posteriorly and receives the great saphenous vein in the inguinal area. After crossing the inguinal ligament it continues as the external iliac vein.

inguinal ligament
A fibrous ligament that extends obliquely from the anterosuperior iliac spine to the pubis and represents the limit between the pelvic and femoral regions. The arteries, veins and nerves of the inferior extremity pass under the crural arch to the thigh.

subcutaneous veins of the anterior face of the thigh
A dense venous network that crosses the knee and the leg just below the skin and carries the venous blood of this area to the great saphenous vein.

pudendal veins
Veins that collect the venous blood from a part of the genitals and terminate in the great saphenous vein near to its union with the femoral vein.

anastomosis of the short and long saphenous veins
When it passes the knee posteriorly, the small saphenous vein terminates in the popliteal vein of the deep venous system, but it also has a communicating branch that unites it with the great saphenous vein.

accessory saphenous vein
The accessory saphenous collects the venous blood from the posterior part of the thigh. It terminates in the superior part of the long saphenous vein.

small saphenous vein
A vein that originates in the external dorsal part of the foot and after passing behind the lateral malleolus of the ankle, reaches the thigh, where it unites with the popliteal vein of the deep venous system. It also has a branch which terminates in the great saphenous vein.

long saphenous vein
A vein that originates in the internal part of the dorsal venous arch of the foot and, after passing in front of the medial malleolus of the ankle, ascends the leg, collecting the venous blood of the subcutaneous venous network of the anterior and internal part of the leg. After passing the knee it reaches the thigh, crossing it superficially in its anterointernal face to terminate in the final portion of the femoral vein.

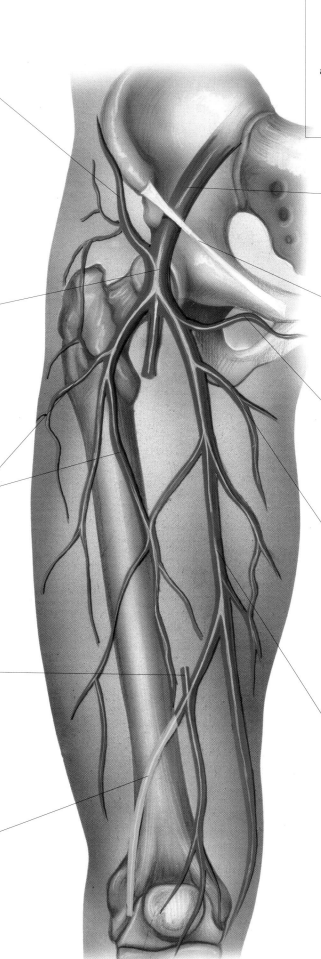

85

THE VENOUS SYSTEM. HAND AND FOREARM. SUPERFICIAL VEINS

VENOUS SYSTEM OF THE SUPERIOR EXTREMITY

The superior and inferior extremities are equipped with twin venous systems, one deep and the other superficial. The deep venous system is a parallel system to the arterial system, with identical names and trajectory, although there are two veins for each artery. For these reasons it is not considered necessary to illustrate it. The superficial venous system, on the contrary, has a different trajectory and nomenclature and runs up the forearm in more superficial areas although it terminates in the deep venous system.

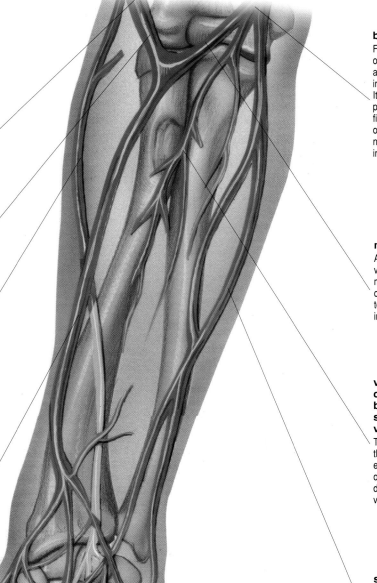

cephalic vein
The cephalic vein originates in the union of the median cephalic vein and the superficial radial vein. It ascends the arm in its external superficial area and terminates in the axillary vein.

median cephalic vein
One of the veins ascends the anterior surface of the flexure of the elbow, from the bifurcation of the median vein to unite with the superficial radial vein to form the cephalic vein.

superficial radial vein
The superficial radial crosses the forearm superficially, firstly posteriorly and subsequently externally. It collects the venous blood from the forearm and also from the external dorsal part of the hand. It unites with the median cephalic vein to form the cephalic vein.

median vein
Vein that ascends the anterior face of the forearm, from the palmar area of the hand to the elbow, where it bifurcates into the median cephalic and median basilic veins. It is joined by various venous branches coming from the anterior face of the forearm.

dorsal venous arch of the hand
The dorsal arch forms the network of veins of the back of the hand, which it collects from the interosseal veins and which it distributes by branches to the radial and ulnar veins.

basilic vein
Formed by the union of the median basilic vein and the superficial ulnar vein in the flexure of the elbow. It then ascends the internal part of the arm to reach the final part of the humeral veins of the deep venous system near to where these terminate in the axillary vein.

median basilic vein
A bifurcation of the median vein, that extends to the medial part of the flexure of the elbow and terminates, together with the ulnar vein, in the basilic vein.

venous communication between the superficial and deep venous systems
Throughout its trajectory, the superficial venous system emits communicating branches or anastomosis with the deep system, to ensure venous return.

superficial ulnar vein
A vein that collects the blood from the medial, dorsal part of the hand, ascends the internal portion of the forearm and terminates, together with the median basilic vein, in the basilic vein.

interosseal veins
Prolongations of the digital veins that terminate in the dorsal venous arch of the hand.

digital veins
The dorsal veins originate in the distal extremes of the fingers and carry the venous blood to the interosseal veins.

86

With Compliments

ark View Gardens - Hendon - London NW4 2PN
020 8202 6776 Fax: 020 8457 4830 Email: rmyers8@btinternet.com
T Reg. No. 702 0418 91

on
ation.com

Compliments copy.

THE VENOUS SYSTEM. ARM AND SHOULDER. SUPERFICIAL VEINS

axillary vein
The vein through which all the
blood from the superficial and deep
venous systems of the superior
extremity is carried to
the subclavian vein. It originates
in the axillary region from the union
of the cephalic and basilic veins of
the superficial system with the
brachial veins of the deep system. It
also receives blood from the
shoulder, scapular, mammary
areas, etc.

**posterior circumflex
humeral vein**
A venous branch that terminates in
the external part of the cephalic vein.
It collects blood from the deltoid
muscle and the shoulder joint.

**anterior circumflex
humeral vein**
A lateral venous branch that
terminates in the cephalic vein and
collects the venous blood from part
of the area of the deltoid muscle.

cephalic vein
The cephalic vein originates
in the union of the median cephalic
vein and the superficial radial vein.
It ascends the arm in its external
superficial area and terminates
in the axillary vein, receiving
venous branches from the
arm and the elbow.

median cephalic vein
One of the veins that ascends
the anterior surface of the flexure
of the elbow, from the
bifurcation of the median vein
to unite with the superficial radial
vein to form the cephalic vein.

superficial radial vein
The superficial radial crosses the
forearm superficially, firstly posteriorly
and subsequently laterally. It collects
venous blood from the forearm
and also from the external dorsal
part of the hand. It unites with
the median cephalic vein to form
the cephalic vein.

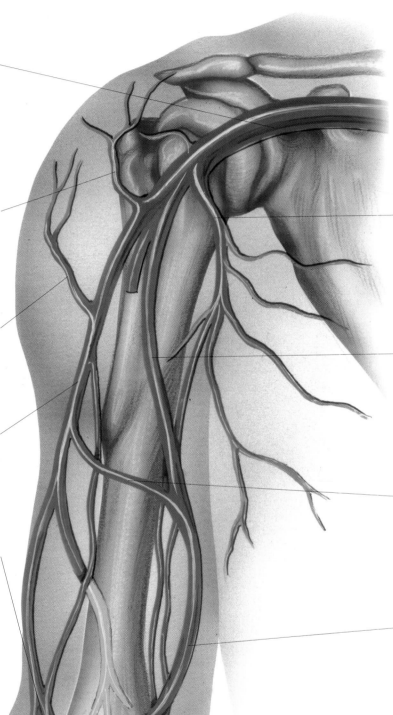

**VENOUS SYSTEM OF
THE SUPERIOR EXTREMITY**

The superior and inferior extremities
are equipped with twin venous systems,
one deep and the other superficial. The deep
venous system is a parallel system to the arterial
system, with identical names and trajectory,
although there are two veins for each artery.
For these reasons it is not considered necessary
to illustrate it. The superficial venous system,
on the contrary, has a different trajectory
and nomenclature and runs up the arm in
more superficial areas although it terminates
in the deep venous system.

thoracic veins
A group of veins that ascend
from the lateral thoracic region
and terminate in the axillary vein.

basilic vein
Formed by the union of the median
basilic vein with the superficial ulnar
vein in the flexure of the elbow. It then
ascends the medial part of the arm to
reach the final part of the brachial veins
of the deep venous system near to where
these terminate in the axillary vein.

**anastomosis of the
cephalic and basilic veins**
The basilic and cephalic veins are united by a
transversal communicating vein or anastomosis,
that allows venous blood to be exchanged
and ensures venous return.

median basilic vein
A bifurcation of the median vein, that
extends to the medial part of the flexure
of the elbow and terminates, together
with the ulnar vein, in the basilic vein.

median vein
Vein that ascends the anterior face of the
forearm, from the palmar area of the hand
to the elbow, where it bifurcates into the
median cephalic and median basilic veins.

superficial ulnar vein
A vein that collects the blood from the
internal, dorsal part of the hand, ascends
the internal portion of the forearm and
terminates, together with the median
basilic vein, in the basilic vein.

87

THE VENOUS SYSTEM. CRANIAL SINUS

superior longitudinal or saggital sinus
A duct that crosses the inside of the cranial vault, from front to back, following a channel excavated in the vault. It collects the venous blood from the orbital area and the internal face of the cerebral hemispheres and terminates in the lateral sinus.

CRANIAL SINUSES
Venous ducts that cross the skull internally through the space adjacent to the dura mater, collecting the venous blood from the brain and the other intracranial organs and carrying it to the internal jugular vein, where they all converge.

straight sinus
The straight sinus collects the venous blood from the base of the brain and a part of the cerebellum. It terminates in the union of the superior longitudinal sinus with the lateral sinus.

posterior occipital sinus
Sinuses that cross the edges of the occipital foramen laterally to reach the termination of the lateral sinuses in the internal jugular vein. They collect the venous blood from the posterior part of the cerebellum.

lateral sinus
The lateral or transverse sinus is born laterally from the union of the superior longitudinal sinus and the straight sinus and, after bordering the sides of the occipital fossa, terminate in the origin of the internal jugular vein.

internal jugular vein
The venous blood collected by the different cranial sinuses is deposited in the internal jugular vein which leaves the skull through the posterior torn hole and continues down the neck.

coronary or intracavernous sinus
An elliptical sinus located within the sella turcica, surrounding the hypophysis gland. It terminates laterally in the coronary sinus.

inferior petrous sinus
The inferior petrous sinuses originate in the cavernous sinuses and terminate in the origin of the internal jugular vein. They cross the inferior part of the petrous bone.

sphenoparietal sinus
The sphenoparietal sinuses cross the sphenoid bone by the posterior edge of the roof of the orbit and terminate in the cavernous sinuses, collecting the venous blood from the anterior area of the brain.

superior petrous sinus
The superior petrous sinuses connect the cavernous sinuses with the lateral sinuses and collect the venous blood from the base of the cerebral hemispheres. They cross the superior part of the petrous bone.

cavernous sinus
The cavernous sinuses are located at each side of the sella turcica where the hypophysis is situated, and collect the blood from the ophthalmic vein, which comes from the orbit, the coronary sinus, and the area of the sphenoid bone. They continue through the petrous sinus.

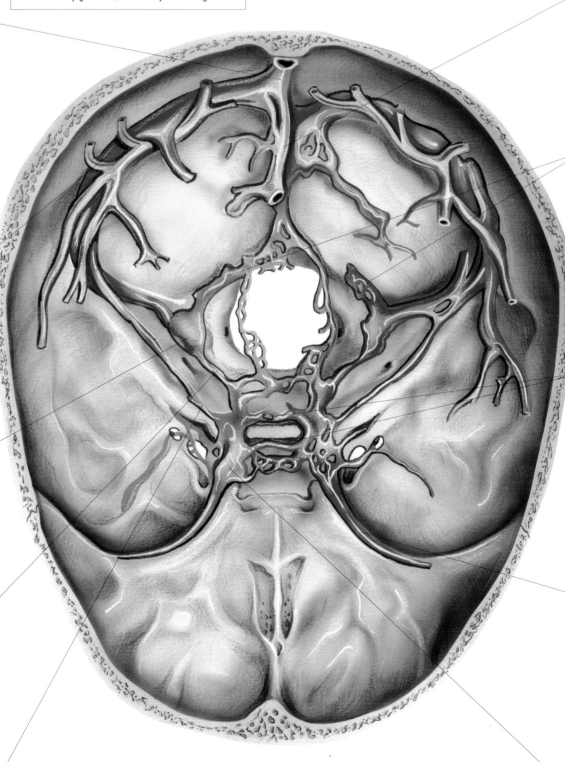

THE VENOUS SYSTEM. NECK AND HEAD

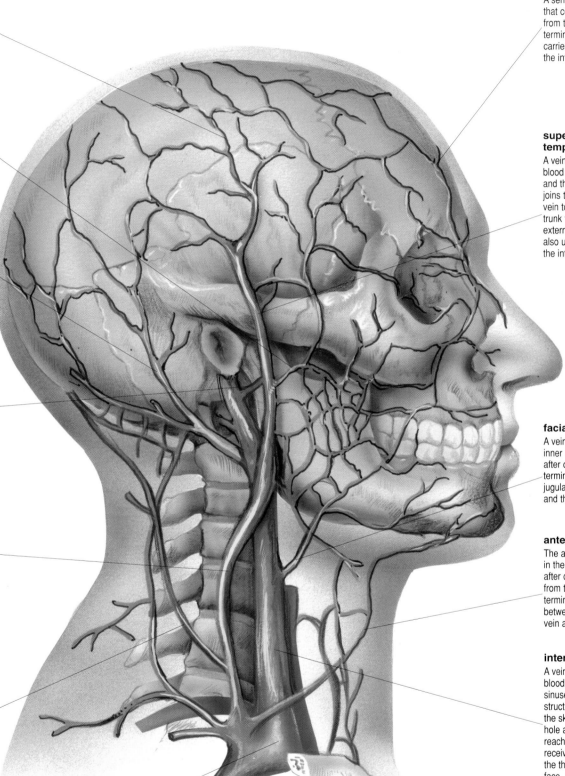

parietal veins
A network of small vessels that collect the venous blood from the parietal area and carry it to the superficial temporal vein.

internal maxillary vein
The internal maxillary collects the venous blood from the maxillary region and unites with the superficial temporal vein, with which it forms a common trunk that terminates in the external jugular vein, also joining with the internal jugular vein, to connect both venous systems.

auricular and occipital veins
They collect the venous blood from the auricular and occipital areas and terminate in the internal jugular vein.

anastomosis between the systems of the external and internal jugular veins
The two main venous systems of the skull are connected by small communicating veins that ensure a correct venous return.

external jugular vein
Vein that crosses the external superficial part of the neck and terminates at the union of the subclavian and internal jugular veins. It originates in the convergence of the veins from the occipital, temporal and maxillary areas and others from the internal jugular system.

vertebral vein
Vein that descends the neck in parallel with the vertebral column and collects the venous blood from that area, terminating together with the external jugular vein in the subclavian vein.

brachiocephalic venous trunk
A common trunk formed by the union of the veins of half of the head (internal jugular) and of the superior extremity (subclavian vein). It terminates in the superior vena cava, which carries the venous blood from both areas to the right atrium of the heart.

frontal veins
A series of small blood vessels that collect the venous blood from the frontal area and terminate in the facial vein that carries the blood to the internal jugular vein.

superficial temporal vein
A vein that collects venous blood from the parietal veins and the temporal area and joins the internal maxillary vein to form a common trunk that terminates in the external jugular vein and is also united to the system of the internal jugular vein.

facial vein
A vein that originates in the inner angle of the eye and, after crossing the facial area, terminates in the internal jugular vein. It has lingual and thyroid branches.

anterior jugular vein
The anterior jugular originates in the submentonian area and, after collecting the venous blood from the anterior area of the neck, terminates close to the union between the external jugular vein and the subclavian vein.

internal jugular vein
A vein that collects the venous blood from the intracranial sinuses, which drain all the structures of the skull. It leaves the skull by the posterior torn hole and descends the neck to reach the brachiocephalic trunk, receiving in its path veins from the thyroid, the tongue, the face, and the temporal area and maxillary areas.

subclavian vein
A vein that comes from the arm and terminates at the brachiocephalic venous trunk. It receives branches from the scapular, thyroid and intercostal area, although many branches go directly to the brachiocephalic trunk.

89

THE VENOUS SYSTEM. ABDOMEN AND PORTAL VEIN

portal vein
The vein that carries the venous blood from the abdominal digestive organs to the liver. It originates in the union of the superior and inferior mesenteric veins and the splenic vein and ascends to the liver, which it enters through the hepatic hilum, dividing into multiple branches inside the liver. In its extrahepatic portion it receives branches from the stomach, gallbladder, the umbilical area and the pancreas.

inferior vena cava
A common trunk that receives the venous blood of the inferior half of the body. It originates in the inferior area of the abdomen from the union of the two common iliac veins (right and left), which collect the blood from the organs of the pelvic cavity and the inferior extremity.

gastric coronary veins
Veins that cross the lesser curvature of the stomach and terminate directly in the portal vein immediately before in enters the hepatic hilum.

splenic vein
The spenic vein originates in the spleen and follows an almost horizontal path to join the inferior and superior mesenteric veins to form the portal vein.

umbilical vein
A vestige of the umbilicus which supplies nutrients to the fetus. After birth, the vein has no function and atrophies.

renal vein
A branch that originates in the renal hilum and carries the venous blood of the kidney to the inferior vena cava which it joins horizontally.

superior mesenteric vein
A vein that transports the venous blood from the small intestine and the right half of the large intestine. It joins with the inferior mesenteric and splenic veins to form the portal vein. It has jejunal, ileocolic, colic, pancreatic and epiploic branches.

gastroepiploic vein
A vein that collects blood from the left border of the stomach and of the omentum which support the intestines. It terminates in the superior mesenteric vein.

right colic vein
The right colic collects blood from the ascending colon and terminates in the superior mesenteric vein.

inferior mesenteric vein
The inferior mesenteric collects the venous blood from the left half of the large intestine. It has hemorrhoidal, sigmoid, rectal and colic branches and joins the splenic vein and posteriorly the superior mesenteric vein to form the portal vein.

common iliac vein
A vein that originates in the union of the internal and external iliac veins and ascends obliquely to join with the opposing common iliac vein to form the inferior vena cava.

genital vein
A venous branch that ascends from the male (testicular vein) and female (ovarian vein) genital organs to terminate in the renal vein.

external iliac vein
A continuation of the femoral vein which collects all the venous blood from the inferior extremity. In the abdomen, it joins the internal iliac vein to form the common iliac vein.

internal iliac vein
Also known as the hypogastric vein. It collects the venous blood of the intrapelvic organs (bladder, uterus, rectum, anus, etc.), of the gluteal area and the external genitals (pudendal veins). It is united to the external iliac vein, and between them they give rise to the common iliac vein.

middle colic vein
A vein that runs alongside the transverse colon, collecting its venous blood and transporting it to the superior mesenteric vein.

left colic vein
A branch that terminates in the inferior mesenteric vein after collecting the venous blood from the descending colon.

THE VENOUS SYSTEM. THORAX, VENA CAVA AND AZYGOS

internal jugular vein
A vein that collects the venous blood from the intracranial sinus, which drains all the structures of the skull. It descends the neck to reach the brachiocephalic trunk. It receives branches from the thyroids, the tongue, the face, the temporal and maxillary areas.

brachiocephalic venous trunk
Two venous trunks whose union gives rise to the superior vena cava. The right trunk receives the venous blood from the right superior extremity and the right half of the head and neck and the left trunk performs a similar function on the opposite side of the body.

vertebral vein
Vein that descends the neck in parallel with the vertebral column and collects the venous blood from that area, terminating together with the external jugular vein in the subclavian vein.

subclavian vein
A continuation of the axillary vein which collects the blood from the superficial and deep venous systems of the superior extremity and joins the internal jugular vein to form the brachiocephalic trunk.

inferior thyroid veins
Veins that collect the venous blood from the inferior part of the thyroid and carry it to the brachiocephalic venous trunk.

superior vena cava
A thick venous trunk that receives all the venous blood of the superior half of the body (trunk, superior extremities and head). It originates in the union of the right and left brachiocephalic trunks and terminates in the right atrium of the heart.

internal mammary vein
A vein which ascends the thoracic wall and terminates in the brachiocephalic trunk near to its union with the superior vena cava. It collects venous blood from the abdomen, diaphragm and anterior intercostal areas.

hemiazygos vein
A vein that runs parallel to the azygos vein on the left border of the vertebral column and collects the venous blood from some intercostal veins. It terminates in the left margin of the azygos vein as a side or double branch at around the eighth and ninth vertebra.

intercostal veins
Venous branches that join the azygos vein horizontally after crossing the intercostal spaces and collecting venous blood from these areas.

azygos vein
Together with the hemiazygos vein, the azygos vein, originating in the thorax, forms a complementary venous system to the vena cava. It collects the venous blood from the mediastinum, the diaphragm, and the intercostal and lumbar areas. It ascends the right side of the vertebral column and terminates in the superior vena cava.

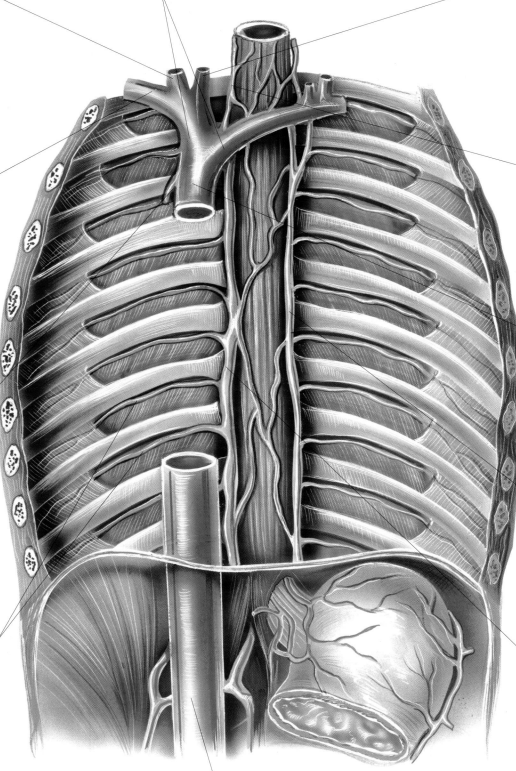

inferior vena cava
A common trunk that receives the venous blood of the inferior half of the body, including the abdomen, pelvis and inferior extremities. After crossing the diaphragm, it enters the thoracic cavity and terminates, together with the superior vena cava, in the right atrium of the heart.

91

DIGESTIVE SYSTEM

▼ GENERAL VIEW

salivary glands
Clusters of glands contained in the walls of the mouth. They secrete the saliva needed to masticate and digest food into the mouth by means of small ducts.

tongue
A flat appendix inside the oral cavity. The front end is free and the back is attached to the anterior zone of the pharynx. It is formed of various muscles which confer a wide range of movements used in swallowing and phonation.

oral cavity
The mouth is responsible for the first steps in digesting the food we eat, including the processes of salivation, mastication and swallowing. The inside of the mouth is lined with a fine layer of mucosa called the buccal mucosa, which extends to the pharynx.

isthmus of the fauces
The narrow passage from the mouth to the pharynx bordered by the soft palate, the base of the tongue and the lateral pillars, where the palatine tonsils are located.

teeth
Bony structures inside the mouth arranged in superior and inferior rows in the gingivae or gums. Their function is to tear and masticate food before it is swallowed.

pharynx
A tube of muscle and membrane that begins in the nasal fossas, descends through the neck and terminates in the oesophagus. It has both respiratory and digestive functions.

oesophagus
A cylindrical duct that extends from the pharynx to the stomach. It descends through the thoracic cavity and diaphragm and has a short section in the abdomen. The walls are formed of muscles which, when contracted, push the food downwards.

cardia
The orifice that connects the stomach with the oesophagus.

pancreas
A glandular organ located behind stomach. Through a small duct called the duct of Wirsung, the pancreas sends secretions, which contain enzymes that aid the digestion of food, to the duodenum.

stomach
The stomach is a large saccular organ that receives food from the oesophagus and stores it during the digestive process. The walls of the stomach contain glands that secrete gastric juices that help break down the food. The contraction of the stomach walls mixes the food within to aid digestion.

92

liver
A large organ located in the right superior angle of the abdomen, in the zone called the right hypochondrium. Its main digestive function is the production of bile, a fluid that is sent to the duodenum through the bile ducts and which is fundamental in the digestion of dietary fats.

ascending colon
The section of the large intestine that ascends the right side of the abdomen vertically from the caecum to the hepatic region.

transverse colon
The section of the large intestine that crosses the abdomen transversally from the hepatic area to the splenic area.

large intestine
The large intestine is a continuation of the small intestine and has a greater diameter. It absorbs water, leaving the unabsorbed remains of food which progressively form the faeces. It has various sections that surround the small intestine.

pylorus
The pylorus is a small, round opening located between the stomach and the duodenum. The surrounding area is called the pyloric region.

descending and sigmoid colon
The section of the large intestine that descends the left side of the abdomen vertically to reach the rectum.

gallbladder
A saccular organ contained with the biliary system which stores the bile produced by the liver until it is sent to the duodenum.

caecum
The initial section of the large intestine, which is formed by a large sac that receives the waste products through the ileocaecal valve.

small intestine
A long tube that leaves the stomach and coils inside the abdominal cavity in multiple angles or intestinal loops. Its function is the digestion, absorption and transport of foods. For better absorption, the internal surfaces are covered with millions of small projections called villi. It consists of three parts, the duodenum, jejunum and ileum.

duodenum
The first section of the small intestine which receives the secretions from the liver and the pancreas.

vermiform appendix
A lymphatic organ attached to the caecum. Its inflammation causes the condition known as appendicitis.

jejunum
The second section of the small intestine.

rectum
The final part of the large intestine, which is a continuation of the sigmoid colon when it enters the pelvic cavity. In its final part it has an expansion called the rectal ampolla which is where the formed faeces are stored until their expulsion.

ileum
The third and final section of the small intestine.

anus
A structure composed of sphincters which forms the final part of the digestive system. By means of a muscular system that consists of two sphincters (internal and external) which can be opened or be closed voluntarily, the anus can expel the faeces.

iliocaecal valve
A valve between the final part of the small intestine, the ileum, and the initial part of the large intestine, the caecum.

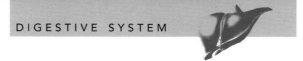

ORAL CAVITY

▼ LATERAL VIEW

vestibule of the mouth
The space between the upper and lower lips and the gingivae.

maxilla
The bone that separates the nasal fossae and the oral cavity and forms part of the hard palate.

buccal mucosa
A fine, rosy membrane that lines all the oral cavity, including the cheeks, the gingivae, the floor of the mouth and the posterior face of the lips. In the tongue it is called the lingual mucosa.

hard palate
The anterior part of the roof of the mouth, which is supported by the maxilla.

soft palate
The posterior part of the roof of the mouth. Its structure of muscle and membrane has no bony support.

nasal pharynx
The superior part of the pharynx which connects with the nasal fossae.

lingual tonsils
Two lymph organs similar to the palatine tonsils, but located behind the tongue.

palatine tonsils
Two round organs located between the anterior and posterior pillars of the veil of the palate. They are lymph organs that form part of the body's defence system.

oral pharynx
The middle part of the pharynx is a tube of muscle and membrane that originates in the nasal fossae and enters the neck. It has respiratory (passage of air) and digestive (passage of food) functions.

teeth
Bony structures inside the mouth arranged in upper and lower rows in the gingivae or gums. Their function is to tear and masticate food before it is swallowed.

tongue
A flat appendix inside the oral cavity. The front end is free and the back is attached to the anterior zone of the pharynx. It is formed of various muscles that confer a wide range of movements used in swallowing and phonation.

laryngeal pharynx
The inferior continuation of the oral pharynx and having the same functions. It constitutes the final part of the pharynx and finishes in a double duct; posteriorly it connects with the oesophagus and anteriorly with the larynx.

mandible
A facial bone that surrounds the oral cavity anteriorly and laterally. Its articulation with the skull is movable, which allows a series of movements that aid mastication and phonation. Various tongue muscles are inserted in the mandible.

hyoid bone
A thin U-shaped bone in which the muscles of the tongue and pharynx are inserted.

epiglottis
A flap of cartilage lying behind the tongue that acts as a cover over the orifice which opens to allow air to pass to the respiratory tract. The epiglottis opens to permit the passage of air and closes when food is being swallowed.

larynx
A tubular formation consisting of cartilaginous structures. It contains membranous folds that form the vocal cords, which allow phonation by vibrating the passing air.

oesophagus
A cylindrical duct that extends from the pharynx to the stomach. The walls are formed of muscles which, when contracted, push the food downwards.

93

THE STRUCTURE OF A TOOTH

root canal
A duct located inside the dental root which carries the blood vessels and nerves to the dental pulp.

crown
The external and visible section of the tooth which emerges from the gum.

neck
The intermediate zone of the tooth located between the crown and the root.

root
The section of the tooth implanted within the gingiva in a cavity called the dental alveolus.

cement
A layer that covers the root of the tooth externally and is equivalent to the enamel of the crown. It is a hard, yellowish substance whose external face corresponds to the periodontal ligament that unites the root with the alveolar bone.

dental alveoli
The dental alveoli are the sockets in the maxilla and mandible in which each of the teeth are implanted.

enamel
The external layer of the crown of the tooth. Whitish in color, the enamel is extremely hard.

dentin
The middle part of the tooth, located between the enamel and the dental pulp. It forms the main structure of the tooth and is very hard.

gingiva
The part of the buccal mucosa that covers the maxilla and mandible in the area of implantation of the teeth.

pulp
The central area of the tooth. It is formed by connective tissue which contains the vascular and nervous terminations.

mandible
The bone in which the lower teeth are implanted.

94

TYPES OF TEETH

incisors
Located in the front part of the gingiva, the incisors have one root and a flat crown. There are four upper and four lower incisors whose function is to bite and tear foods.

canines
The canine teeth are located behind the incisors. They have a sole root and a conical, pointed crown. There two upper and two lower canines whose function is to tear and bite food.

premolars
Located behind the canines, the premolars have a single root and a cubical crown. There are four upper and four lower premolars whose function is to crush and grind food.

molars
The molars are located at the back of the mouth behind the premolars. They have multiple roots and an irregularly shaped crown. People have as many as six upper and six lower molars, although some people lack the last two upper and lower molars on each side, the wisdom teeth. Their function is to crush and to grind food.

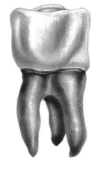

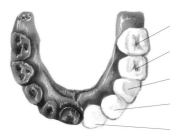
TEETHING

1ST TEETHING

Deciduous dentition. Babies are normally born without teeth, which begin to appear after about six months. The first set of teeth, the deciduous dentition, is temporary and will fall out spontaneously as the child grows, to be replaced by the permanent teeth. There are usually 20 deciduous teeth.

APPROXIMATE AGE OF ERUPTION

upper central incisor 8–10 months

upper lateral incisor 9–12 months

upper canine 18–24 months

first upper premolar 13–15 months

second upper premolar 24–30 months

alveoli
Cavities inside the mandible and maxilla which contain the dental buds until their eruption.

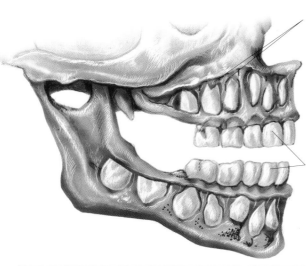

second lower premolar 24–30 months

first lower premolar 13–15 months

lower canine 18–24 months

lower lateral incisor 9–12 months

lower central incisor 6–9 months

deciduous dentition
Temporary teething which begins to emerge at around six months and is complete by twenty-four to thirty months. The deciduous teeth begin to fall out spontaneously after about six years of age.

2ND TEETHING

Permanent teething or second teething. It begins to erupt around six years of age when the deciduous dentition begins to fall out, although it is often not completed until adulthood. Normally, adults have 32 permanent upper and lower teeth

APPROXIMATE AGE OF ERUPTION

upper central incisor 6–8 years

upper lateral incisor 6–8 years

upper canine 11–12 years

first upper premolar 10–11 years

second upper premolar 12–13 years

first upper molar 6–7 years

second upper molar 12–14 years

third upper molar 18–30 years
(In some people it may not erupt).

third lower molar 18–30 years
(In some people it may not erupt).

second lower molar 12–14 years

first lower molar 6–7 years

second lower premolar 10–11 years

first lower premolar 12–13 years

lower canine 11–12 years

lower lateral incisor 8–9 years

lower central incisor 8–9 years

95

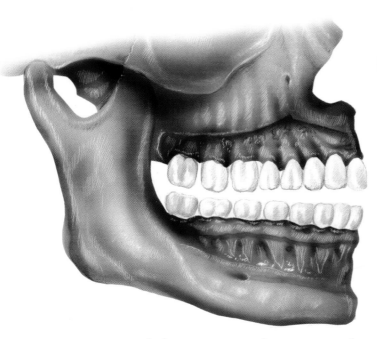

incisors	canine	premolars	molar

   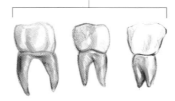

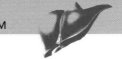

THE OESOPHAGUS

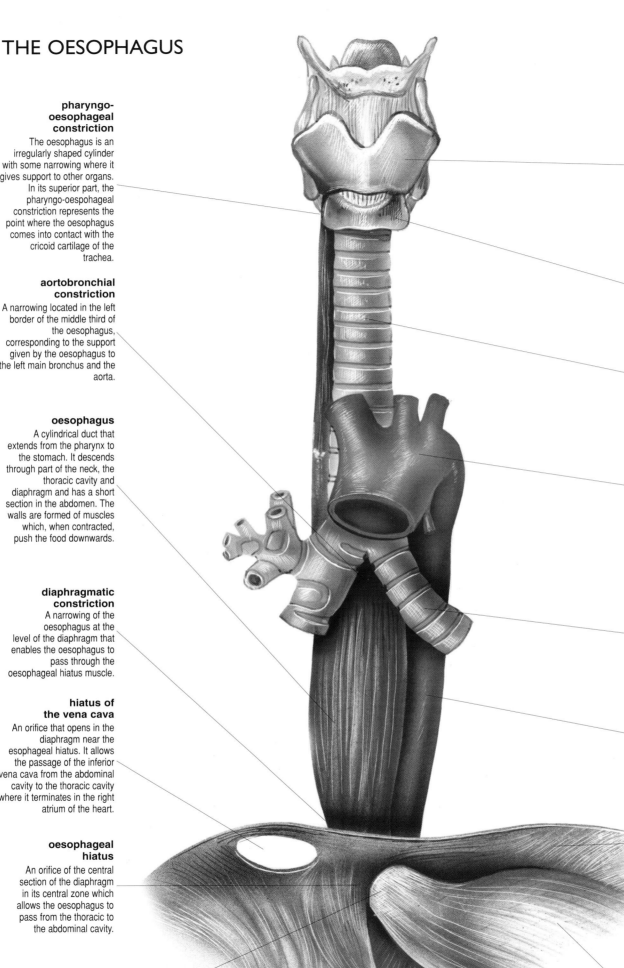

pharyngo-oesophageal constriction
The oesophagus is an irregularly shaped cylinder with some narrowing where it gives support to other organs. In its superior part, the pharyngo-oespohageal constriction represents the point where the oesophagus comes into contact with the cricoid cartilage of the trachea.

aortobronchial constriction
A narrowing located in the left border of the middle third of the oesophagus, corresponding to the support given by the oesophagus to the left main bronchus and the aorta.

oesophagus
A cylindrical duct that extends from the pharynx to the stomach. It descends through part of the neck, the thoracic cavity and diaphragm and has a short section in the abdomen. The walls are formed of muscles which, when contracted, push the food downwards.

diaphragmatic constriction
A narrowing of the oesophagus at the level of the diaphragm that enables the oesophagus to pass through the oesophageal hiatus muscle.

hiatus of the vena cava
An orifice that opens in the diaphragm near the esophageal hiatus. It allows the passage of the inferior vena cava from the abdominal cavity to the thoracic cavity where it terminates in the right atrium of the heart.

oesophageal hiatus
An orifice of the central section of the diaphragm in its central zone which allows the oesophagus to pass from the thoracic to the abdominal cavity.

cardia
The opening between the oesophagus and stomach which acts as a sphincter as or valve, opening to admit food and closing to prevent a reflux.

thyroid cartilage
A cartilage that forms the anterior wall of the larynx. Its anterior part marks a protuberance in the neck known as the Adam's apple, which is more pronounced in males.

cricoid cartilage
A cartilaginous ring that forms the inferior limit of the larynx and is supported by the superior part of the oesophagus.

trachea
A tubular structure that forms part of the respiratory system and descends in parallel and anterior to the oesophagus to connect the larynx with the lungs.

arch of the aorta
The aorta ascends from the left ventricle and then immediately curves left and descends, forming an arch located anterior to the superior section of the oesophagus.

left main bronchus
One of the two main bronchi into which the trachea bifurcates. The left bronchus is supported by the middle section of the oesophagus.

thoracic aorta
Continuation of the arch of the aorta, which descends posteriorly and in parallel with the oesophagus through the diaphragm.

diaphragm
A flat muscle that separates the thoracic and abdominal cavities. It has various orifices or hiatuses that allow organs such as the oesophagus and aorta to pass from one cavity to another.

stomach
A large saccular organ. The oesophagus passes through the diaphragm and deposits its contents in the stomach after entering the abdomen. The stomach accumulates the ingested food and begins to digest it through the action of the gastric juices secreted by the glands of the walls of the stomach.

96

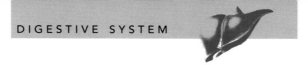

STOMACH

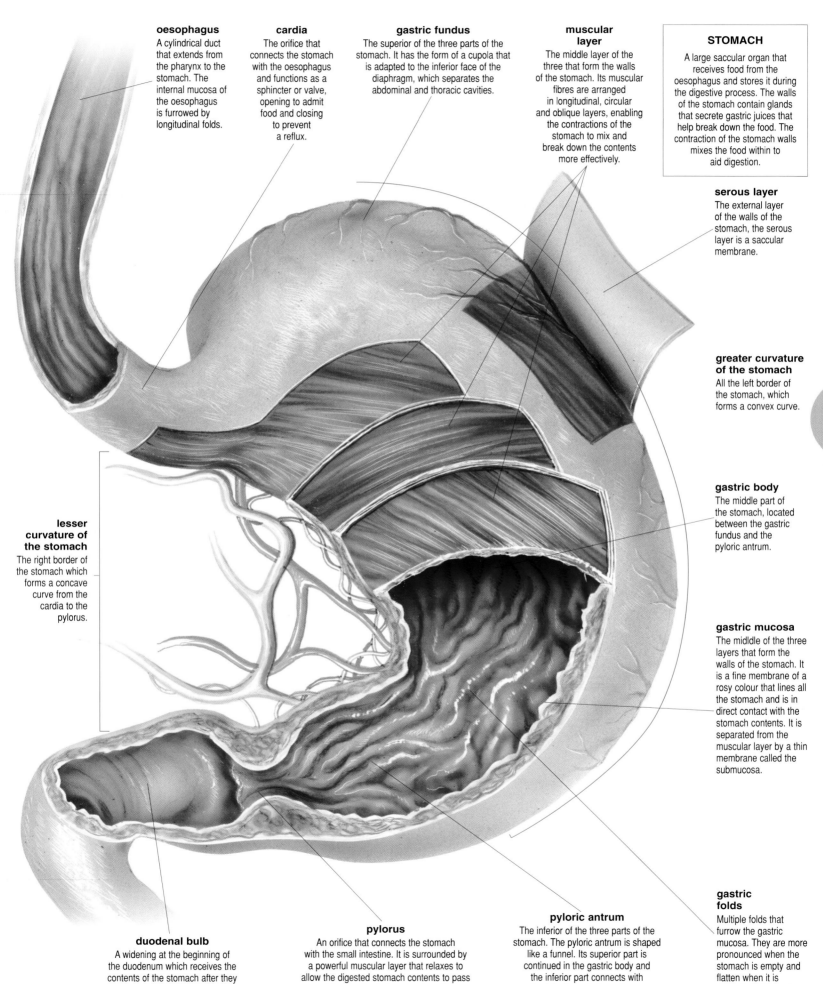

oesophagus
A cylindrical duct that extends from the pharynx to the stomach. The internal mucosa of the oesophagus is furrowed by longitudinal folds.

cardia
The orifice that connects the stomach with the oesophagus and functions as a sphincter or valve, opening to admit food and closing to prevent a reflux.

gastric fundus
The superior of the three parts of the stomach. It has the form of a cupola that is adapted to the inferior face of the diaphragm, which separates the abdominal and thoracic cavities.

muscular layer
The middle layer of the three that form the walls of the stomach. Its muscular fibres are arranged in longitudinal, circular and oblique layers, enabling the contractions of the stomach to mix and break down the contents more effectively.

STOMACH
A large saccular organ that receives food from the oesophagus and stores it during the digestive process. The walls of the stomach contain glands that secrete gastric juices that help break down the food. The contraction of the stomach walls mixes the food within to aid digestion.

serous layer
The external layer of the walls of the stomach, the serous layer is a saccular membrane.

greater curvature of the stomach
All the left border of the stomach, which forms a convex curve.

97

gastric body
The middle part of the stomach, located between the gastric fundus and the pyloric antrum.

lesser curvature of the stomach
The right border of the stomach which forms a concave curve from the cardia to the pylorus.

gastric mucosa
The midldle of the three layers that form the walls of the stomach. It is a fine membrane of a rosy colour that lines all the stomach and is in direct contact with the stomach contents. It is separated from the muscular layer by a thin membrane called the submucosa.

gastric folds
Multiple folds that furrow the gastric mucosa. They are more pronounced when the stomach is empty and flatten when it is distended with food.

pyloric antrum
The inferior of the three parts of the stomach. The pyloric antrum is shaped like a funnel. Its superior part is continued in the gastric body and the inferior part connects with the intestines via the pylorus.

pylorus
An orifice that connects the stomach with the small intestine. It is surrounded by a powerful muscular layer that relaxes to allow the digested stomach contents to pass and then contracts to prevent a reflux.

duodenal bulb
A widening at the beginning of the duodenum which receives the contents of the stomach after they pass through the pylorus.

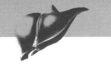

SMALL AND LARGE INTESTINES

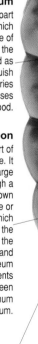

SMALL INTESTINE

A long tube of more than six metres in length that coils inside the abdominal cavity in multiple angles or intestinal folds. It continues the process of digesting and absorbing the stomach contents and consists of three parts: the duodenum, jejunum and ileum.

hepatic flexure of the colon

An angle formed by the colon at the level of the liver which serves as the limit of the ascending colon and the transverse colon.

transverse colon

The section of the large intestine that crosses the abdomen transversally from the hepatic area to the splenic area and continues as the descending colon.

splenic flexure of the colon

An angle formed by the colon at the level of the spleen which marks the limit between the transverse and descending colon.

LARGE INTESTINE

The large intestine is a continuation of the small intestine, which it surrounds like a frame. It absorbs water, leaving the unabsorbed remains of food which progressively form the faeces. It has various sections; the caecum, ascending colon, transverse colon, descending colon, sigmoid colon and the rectum.

duodenum

The first part of the small intestine, which a forms a large C that surrounds the head of the pancreas. It consists of three parts: the first is oblique and begins as the pylorus, the second is descending and the third is ascending and terminates in the angle of Treitz to give way to the jejunum. The duodenum receives the secretions of the liver and pancreas which aid the digestive process.

jejunum

The second or middle part of the small intestine, which begins at the angle of Treitz. The union with the ileum is not well defined as there is little to distinguish them. The jejunum carries out most of the processes of absorption of food.

íleon

The third and final part of the small intestine. It connects with the large intestine through a sphincter muscle known as the ileocecal valve or Bauhin's valve, which allows the contents of the intestine to pass to the large intestine and prevents reflux. The ileum absorbs many nutrients that have not been absorbed in the duodenum and the jejunum.

descending colon

The section of the large intestine that descends the left side of the abdomen vertically to reach the rectum.

sigmoid colon

A continuation of the descending colon which enters the pelvic cavity. Its shape varies from one person to another.

rectum

The final part of the large intestine. In its final part it has an expansion called the rectal ampolla which is where the formed faeces are stored until their expulsion.

ascending colon

A duct that ascends the right side of the abdomen vertically from the caecum to reach the hepatic region, where it forms an angle and continues as the transverse colon.

caecum

The Initial part of the large intestine, which is formed by a large sac that receives the contents of the small intestine through the ileocaecal valve or Bauhin's valve.

vermiform appendix

A lymphatic organ attached to the cecum. Its inflammation causes the condition known as appendicitis.

anus

A sphincter or valve which is the final part of the digestive tract. It contracts or relaxes voluntarily allowing the expulsion of faeces.

LARGE INTESTINE. THE CAECUM AND ANAL AREA

taenia of the colon
The colon is bordered by three taeniae, the free, omental and mesocolic taeniae which serve as insertion membranes of the peritoneum.

haustra
Saccular dilations or semi-lunar crests that correspond to the interior constrictions or folds of the large intestine.

ileum
The third and final part of the small intestine. It connects with the large intestine through the ileocecal valve or Bauhin's valve, which allows the contents of the intestine to pass to the large intestine and prevents reflux.

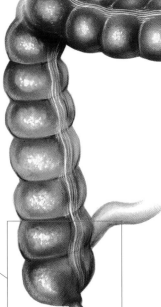

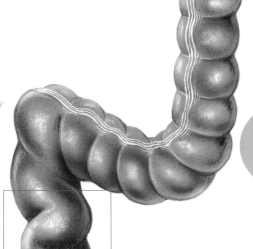

CAECUM

ANAL AREA

semilunar folds or crests
Transverse constrictions that cover all the circumference of the interior surface of the large intestine. Externally they appear as the haustra or semi-lunar crests.

caecum
The initial part of the large intestine, located in the right inferior abdomen, in the right iliac fossa. It is saccular and is also known as the caecal ampulla. It receives and stores the contents of the ileum.

vermiform appendix
A cylindrical lymphatic organ that hangs from the caecum to which it is connected by a small orifice. Its walls are covered by abundant mucosal glands and lymphatic tissue.

ileocaecal valve
An oval orifice, also called Bauhin's valve, which connects the ileum (small intestine) with the caecum (large intestine).

semilunar valves
Small half-moon-shaped folds that surround the anus at the point where it joins the rectum.

rectum
The final part of the large intestine. In its final part it has an expansion called the rectal ampolla which is where the formed faeces are stored until their expulsion.

hemorrhoidal veins
An abundant network of veins that surround the anal canal. When they undergo sustained pressure, they become enlarged and dilated causing the appearance of dilations known as haemorrhoids.

anal folds
Radial folds that surround the final part of the anal duct. When the anus is contracted they are more pronounced, but may disappear when the anus is open, and are relaxed during defaecation.

internal anal sphincter
A ring of smooth muscular fibres located in the interior of the anal orifice. It opens and closes involuntarily, depending on the amount of faeces in the rectum. When the rectum is full, the sphincter opens, producing the desire to defecate.

external anal sphincter
A ring of striated muscular fibres surrounding the exterior of the anal orifice. It can be contracted or relaxed voluntarily when the individual perceives the desire to defecate, allowing control of the process of defecation.

anus
A tubular structure that connects the alimentary canal with the exterior to allow the expulsion of the faecal bolus.

STRUCTURE OF THE STOMACH WALLS AND INTESTINES

mucous layer
The mucous layer lines the stomach and is formed by multiple protuberances and depressions. It contains secretory glands that produce digestive enzymes, hydrochloric acid, bicarbonate, water and mucous substances.

submucous layer
A very thin layer rich in nervous and vascular terminations.

muscular layer
A thick layer of muscle formed of three layers of flat muscle fibres arranged in longitudinal, circular and oblique fashion. When contracted they move in such a way as to mix the stomach contents.

adventitia
The outermost layer of connective tissue that surrounds the sac of the stomach and forms part of the peritoneal sac.

STOMACH

100

mucous layer
The mucous layer lines the small intestine internally. It is covered by tiny intestinal villi and contains multiple secretory glands which produce digestive enzymes and mucous substances that protect the mucosa from the chlorhydric acid of the stomach.

SMALL INTESTINE

muscular layer
A layer formed of smooth muscle fibres arranged in a longitudinal and circular formation.

submucous layer
A very thin layer rich in nervous and vascular terminations.

adventitia
The outermost layer of connective tissue that surrounds the small intestine and contains blood vessels.

muscular layer
A muscular layer formed of flat muscle fibres arranged longitudinally and circularly. The longitudinal fibres do not surround the intestine but are grouped together to form the taenia, a thin layer of longitudinal muscle.

LARGE INTESTINE

mucous layer
The mucous layer lines the internal surface of the large intestine. It is much smoother than the corresponding layer in the small intestine and is formed of flat elevations that contain multiple secretory glands that produce mucous substances.

submucous layer
A very thin layer rich in nervous and vascular terminations.

adventitia
The outermost layer of connective tissue that surrounds the large intestine and contains blood vessels.

THE PERITONEUM

coronary ligament
The largest of the ligaments forming the peritoneal membranes that cover the superior part of the liver and unite it with the diaphragm. The extreme sections of the coronary ligament are known as the right and left triangular ligaments.

falciform ligament
The falciform ligament connects the anterior and superior faces of the liver to the anterior abdominal wall and diaphragm.

spleen
An oval organ located in the left superior angle of the abdomen, in the left hypochondrium. It is posterior to the stomach and united to it by a peritoneal ligament called the gastrosplenic omentum. It is a lymph organ that stores and replenishes the blood cells.

liver
The liver is attached to the lesser omentum, peritoneal membranes which, in their superior part join to form a series of ligaments which attach the liver to the diaphragm.

gastrosplenic omentum
A membrane that joins the superior part of the greater curvature of the stomach with the hilum of the spleen.

stomach
The anterior and posterior face of the stomach are covered by the serous membranes of the peritoneum, which continue upwards to form the lesser omentum that attaches it to the liver, and downwards to form the greater omentum.

101

gallbladder
A saccular organ forming part of the system of the hepatic excretory or biliary system. It stores and concentrates the bile produced by the liver until it is sent to the duodenum.

gastrohepatic omentum
Also known as the lesser omentum, this is a membrane that attaches the lesser curvature of the stomach to the inferior face of the liver.

gastrocolic omentum
Also known as the greater omentum. A membrane that unites the inferior part of the stomach with the transverse colon. In addition, the membrane of the omentum forms a layer overlying the transversal colon and small intestine.

descending colon
The posterior surface of the descending colon is directly attached to the abdominal wall, and the rest is covered by the peritoneum. In its final part, a ligament attaches it to the wall of the pelvic cavity.

ascending colon
Also known as the right colon. It is only covered by the peritoneum in its anterior surface, as the posterior is attached directly to the abdominal wall, making this part of the colon slightly mobile.

small intestine
The anterior separation of the folds of the jejunum and the ileum reveals the mesentery, which supports the folds and attaches them to the posterior abdominal wall.

PERITONEUM
A saccular membrane that surrounds a large part of the abdominal organs, some completely. It consists of two layers: the parietal peritoneum, which is attached to the walls of the abdominal cavity, and the visceral peritoneum, which is introduced between the viscera and surrounds and attaches them. Intraperitoneal organs include the stomach, the spleen, the small intestine and almost all of the large intestine.

mesentery
Part of the peritoneum that supports the folds of the small intestine and attaches them to the posterior wall of the abdomen. It contains numerous blood vessels and nerves.

transverse colon
The anterior and posterior transverse colon is covered by the peritoneum. The membranes join to form the greater omentum in its superior part. The posterior face contains a membranous partition called the transverse mesocolon that unites it to the peritoneal layer that covers the posterior wall of the abdomen.

THE LIVER

common hepatic duct
A duct that carries bile from the hepatic hilum. After a short extrahepatic section it joins the cystic duct coming from the gallbladder to form the common bile duct.

coronary ligament
A membrane that unites the superior part of the liver with the diaphragm.

hepatic fissure
A large sulcus that divides the liver externally and internally into two segments or lobes.

inferior vena cava
A thick, venous trunk that collects the blood from the inferior extremities and the abdominal organs and carries it to the right atrium of the heart. The suprahepatic veins, which carry blood from the liver, join the vena cava posterior to the liver.

LIVER
A large organ located in the right superior angle of the abdomen, in the zone called the right hypochondrium. Its main digestive function is the production of bile, a fluid that is sent to the duodenum through the biliary ducts and which is fundamental in the digestion of dietary fats. The liver is vital in producing energy for the body as it converts a large part of the glucose and other nutrients absorbed into usable energy.

capsule of Gibson
An external layer formed of fibrous tissue that covers all the liver. It has a red-brown colour and a granular aspect.

intrahepatic ducts
The interior of the liver contains small ducts that converge in the hepatic hilum and form the common hepatic duct. Their function is to collect and transport the bile secretions.

left hepatic lobe
The liver is divided into two segments or lobes, of which the left or internal lobe is the smaller.

right hepatic lobe
The liver is divided into two segments or lobes, of which the right or external lobe is the largest.

spleen
An oval organ located in the left superior angle of the abdomen, in the left hypochondrium.

cystic duct
A thin duct that leaves the gallbladder and joins with the common hepatic duct to form the common bile duct.

hepatic hilum
An orifice located in the inferior face of the liver through which the hepatic veins and arteries and the common hepatic duct pass.

gallbladder
A saccular organ contained with the biliary system which stores and concentrates the bile produced by the liver until it is sent to the duodenum.

abdominal aorta
Part of the aorta that descends the abdomen vertically. It branches into a thick artery called the coeliac trunk which, in turn, branches into the hepatic artery.

common bile duct
A duct formed by the union of the cystic and common hepatic ducts. The bile, together with the pancreatic secretions, is emptied into the duodenum through the major duodenal papilla or papilla of Vater.

coeliac trunk
A thick, arterial trunk that originates from the abdominal aorta and has branches to the liver, stomach and spleen.

portal vein
A thick, venous trunk that enters the liver through the hepatic hilum. It is formed by the union of the superior and inferior mesenteric veins, which collect the venous blood from the large and small intestines, and the splenic vein, which collects blood from the spleen.

stomach
A large saccular organ located in the superior part of the abdomen, in the epigastric region and behind and below the liver.

duodenum
The first part of the small intestine going from the stomach to the jejunum. It receives the secretions of the liver and pancreas which enter through the major duodenal papilla or papilla of Vater.

main pancreatic duct or duct of Wirsung
A duct that carries the pancreatic secretions from the pancreas to the duodenum which it enters through the major duodenal papilla jointly with the common bile duct.

pancreas
A glandular organ located below the liver and behind the stomach. It produces the pancreatic juices that go to the duodenum to aid the digestion of foods. In addition, it manufactures a hormone called insulin which enters the bloodstream and is fundamental in the metabolism of sugars.

hepatic artery
A branch of the coeliac trunk that enters the liver through the hepatic hilum, forming branches in its interior. It supplies the liver with arterial blood. (In the drawing, the artery is displaced downwards to show the portal vein and common hepatic duct).

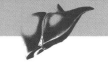
STRUCTURE OF THE LIVER

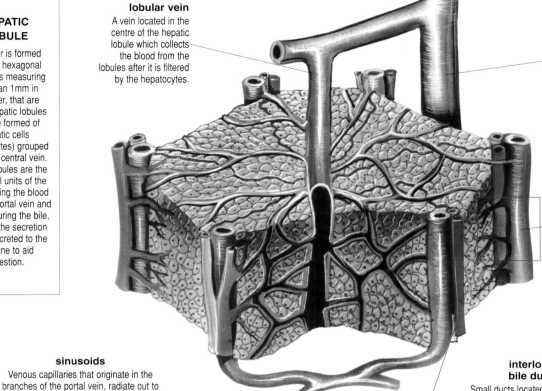

HEPATIC LOBULE

The liver is formed of small hexagonal structures measuring less than 1mm in diameter, that are called hepatic lobules and are formed of hepatic cells (hepatocytes) grouped around a central vein. These lobules are the functional units of the liver, filtering the blood from the portal vein and manufacturing the bile, which is the secretion that is excreted to the intestine to aid digestion.

central lobular vein

A vein located in the centre of the hepatic lobule which collects the blood from the lobules after it is filtered by the hepatocytes.

sublobular vein

The sublobular veins are located between the lobules. They collect the blood from the central lobular veins and converge to form the suprahepatic veins that carry the blood from the liver to the inferior vena cava.

periportal space

The space between the hepatic lobules, through which the branches of the portal vein, the hepatic artery and the interlobular bile ducts pass. This space is surrounded by the conjunctive tissue that encloses the hepatic lobules.

sinusoids

Venous capillaries that originate in the branches of the portal vein, radiate out to the hepatic lobule and take the venous blood to the hepatocytes, where it is filtered and the substances needed by the hepatocytes are extracted. The sinusoids terminate in a vein located in the centre of the hepatic lobule that is called the central lobular vein.

interlobular bile ductule

Small ducts located in the periphery of the hepatic lobule, which collect the bile transported by the biliary canaliculi. The interlobular bile ductules converge to form thicker biliary ducts which terminate in the large right and left intrahepatic ducts, which carry the bile out of the liver.

branch of the portal vein

The portal vein carries the venous blood to the liver. Inside the liver, it branches into successive ramifications that surround the hepatic lobule and carry the blood to it.

103

Kuppfer's cells

Kuppfer's cells are lymphoid cells contained within the sinusoids whose function is to neutralize any foreign bodies that could damage the body, such as bacteria, dead cells, etc.

biliary canaliculus

A thin duct that runs between the hepatocytes and collects the bile that these secrete, transporting it to the interlobular bile ducts.

hepatocytes

The cells that form the hepatic tissue. They perform the many complex functions of the liver, such as the storage of glycogen to provide the body's glucose reserve, the manufacture of proteins or the filtration of the blood to produce bile.

branch of the hepatic artery

The hepatic artery carries arterial blood to the liver. Inside the liver, the hepatic artery branches successively to reach the periphery of the hepatic lobule, contributing the blood necessary for the operation of the hepatocytes. This blood is then excreted to the sinusoids where it is mixed with the venous blood.

THE GALLBLADDER

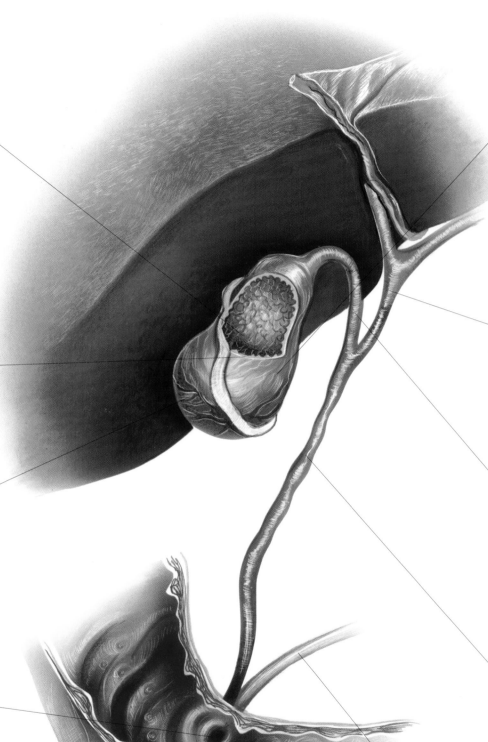

mucous layer
The internal layer of the three that form the wall of the gallbladder. It covers the internal surface of the gallbladder and is furrowed by numerous folds. It contains glands that produce mucous substances.

muscular layer
The central of the three layers that form the wall of the gallbladder. It is composed of muscular fibres that, when contracted, cause the bile accumulated in the gallbladder to be expelled through the cystic duct.

serous layer
The external of the three layers of the wall of the gallbladder. It is formed by the prolongation of the peritoneal membranes that cover the liver.

major duodenal papilla or **papilla of Vater**
An orifice that is the termination of the short common canal of the extrahepatic biliary tree and the pancreatic ducts or ducts of Wirsung, and through which they excrete their secretions into the duodenum.The ducts unite to form a small widening which is called the ampulla of Vater.

duodenum
The second part of the small intestine going from the stomach to the jejunum. It receives the secretions of the liver and pancreas which enter through the major duodenal papilla or papilla of Vater.

gallbladder
A saccular organ contained within the biliary system which stores and concentrates the bile produced by the liver until it is sent to the duodenum. It is attached to the inferior face of the liver and consists of a part near the cystic duct, called the neck of the gallbladder, a central part called the body and a distal part called the floor of the gallbladder.

common hepatic duct
A duct that carries bile from the hepatic hilum and which results from the union of the right and left intrahepatic ducts. After a short extrahepatic section it joins the cystic duct coming from the gallbladder to form the common bile duct.

cystic duct
A thin duct that leaves the gallbladder and joins with the common hepatic duct to form the common bile duct. Bile is transported through the cystic duct to the gallbladder, where it is stored and concentrated, before its expulsion. The valves it contains may give it a rosy aspect.

common bile duct
A duct formed by the union of the cystic and common hepatic ducts. The bile, together with the pancreatic secretions, is emptied into the duodenum through the major duodenal papilla or papilla of Vater. In its termination, it presents, as does the main pancreatic duct, a small muscular sphincter that only opens when the pancreatic fluids are needed.

main pancreatic duct or **duct of Wirsung**
A duct that carries the pancreatic secretions from the pancreas to the duodenum which it enters through the major duodenal papilla jointly with the common bile duct. In its termination, it presents, as does the common bile duct, a small muscular sphincter which only opens when the pancreatic fluids are needed.

PANCREAS

gallbladder
A saccular organ contained with the biliary system which stores and concentrates the bile produced by the liver until it is sent to the duodenum.

cystic duct
A thin duct that leaves the gallbladder and joins with the common hepatic duct to form the common bile duct.

common bile duct
A duct formed by the union of the cystic and common hepatic ducts. The bile, together with the pancreatic secretions, is emptied into the duodenum through the major duodenal papilla or papilla of Vater.

common hepatic duct
A duct which carries the bile from the liver. After a short extrahepatic passage, it joins the cystic duct coming from the gallbladder to form the common bile duct.

main pancreatic duct or of Wirsung
A duct that carries the pancreatic secretions produced by the secretory sacs called acini from the pancreas to the duodenum, which it enters through the major duodenal papilla or papilla of Vater.

coeliac trunk
A thick, arterial trunk that originates in the abdominal aorta and has branches to the liver, stomach and spleen, which in turn branch into the pancreatic arteries.

PANCREAS
A glandular organ with various functions. The pancreas manufactures the pancreatic juices that go to the duodenum to aid the digestion of food. It also manufactures a hormone called insulin that is sent to the blood and is essential for the metabolism of sugars. The digestive function of the pancreas is carried out by multiple secretory sacs called acini. The pancreas is composed of three sections, the head, body and tail.

second portion of the duodenum
The second of the three portions of the duodenum descends vertically. It contains the papillae where the main bile duct from the liver and the main and accessory pancreatic ducts terminate.

smaller papilla of the duodenum
A small eminence in whose vertex a small orifice opens to allow the accessory pancreatic duct or duct of Santorini to reach the duodenum.

accessory pancreatic duct or duct of Santorini
A small duct that originates in the main pancreatic duct and terminates in the duodenum through the smaller papilla, excreting pancreatic secretions into the small intestine.

major duodenal papilla or papilla of Vater
An orifice that is the termination of the short common canal of the extrahepatic biliary tree and the pancreatic duct or duct of Wirsung, and through which they excrete their secretions into the duodenum. The ducts unite to form a small widening called the ampulla of Vater.

head of the pancreas
The most voluminous part of the pancreas, located between the three sections of the duodenum, which contains the two ducts that end in the duodenum.

superior mesenteric vein
A large vein that collects the venous blood from the small intestine and a part of the large intestine and also from the pancreas when it passes behind it.

105

tail of the pancreas
The thinner, superior end of the pancreas which has a flat, slightly pointed shape.

body of the pancreas
The central part of the pancreas which extends from the head, to which it is united by the narrower neck of the pancreas, to the tail.

third portion of the duodenum
The last of the three sections of the duodenum follows a slightly ascending horizontal path to terminate in the flexure called the angle of Treitz, which marks the beginning of the jejunum.

superior mesenteric artery
A branch of the abdominal aorta that passes behind the pancreas. Its branches supply part of the pancreas, the small intestine and a part of the large intestine.

THE RESPIRATORY SYSTEM

▼ GENERAL VIEW

nasal fossae
The cavities forming the initial part of the respiratory system, through which the air is inspired and expired. As it passes through the nasal fossae, the air is filtered and warmed to aid correct respiration.

nasal pharynx
The nasal fossae end at the nasal pharynx which is the upper part of a larger duct called the pharynx, which has both digestive and respiratory functions, although in the nasal pharynx they are mainly respiratory.

oral pharynx
The central portion of the pharynx, which is located immediately behind the oral cavity. It has both digestive and respiratory functions, ingesting food and inspiring and expiring air.

laryngeal pharynx
The lower part of the pharynx, which communicates directly with the prolongation of the digestive system (oesophagus) and with the inferior respiratory tract (larynx), sharing functions with both systems.

carina
The area in which the trachea bifurcates into the two main bronchi.

pulmonary hila
The lungs have internal openings called pulmonary hila through which the pulmonary bronchi and blood vessels enter.

superior lobe of the right lung
The superior lobe occupies the superior half of the right lung.

middle lobe of the right lung
The middle lobe is located in the middle and anteromedial area of the right lung.

inferior lobe of the right lung
The inferior lobe is located in the most inferior and lateral portion of the right lung.

horizontal fissure
A sulcus that separates the superior lobe from the middle lobe.

oblique fissure of the right lung
A sulcus that separates the middle lobe from the inferior lobe of the lung.

epiglottis
A cartilaginous structure that acts as a cover for the orifice of the inferior respiratory tract. When open, it allows air to enter or leave. When shut, it protects the respiratory system from the entrance of food. The epiglottis is located at the posterior base of the tongue and its movements are controlled by powerful muscles.

glottis
Also known as the vestibule of the larynx, the glottis is the cavity giving entry to the larynx, and is located immediately underneath the epiglottis.

larynx
A tubular duct formed of cartilaginous structures that contain membranous folds known as the vocal cords, whose vibrations as the air passes permit phonation.

trachea
The inferior prolongation of the larynx, with the same tubular shape. It is formed of a series of cartilaginous rings. Its function is to allow the inspired and expired air to pass, filtering it through a mucous layer containing prolongations or cilia and secretory mucous glands.

superior lobe of the left lung
The superoanterior portion of the left lung.

inferior lobe of the left lung
The inferoposterior portion of the left lung.

right and left main bronchi
The final part of the trachea bifurcates to form two lateral ducts called the right and left main bronchi, which have the same tubular form and cartilaginous structure. After a brief extrapulmonary section, the two bronchi enter the lungs.

oblique fissure of the left lung
A fissure that separates the superior and inferior lobes of the left lung.

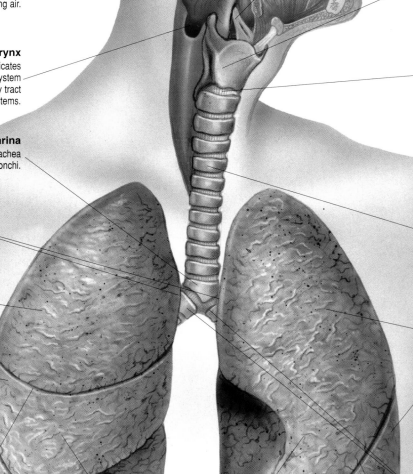

lungs
Two organs formed of spongy, connective tissue located on either side of the thoracic cavity, supported by the diaphragm. They contain the bronchi, bronchioles, alveoli and blood vessels involved in respiration. The lungs are covered by a layer known as the pleura.

106

THE UPPER AIRWAY

▼ LATERAL VIEW

conchae
Bony protuberances covered by nasal mucosa located in the lateral walls of the nasal fossae. They create turbulence in the inspired air, warming and humidifying it before it reaches the pharynx.

paranasal sinuses
Cavities located in the frontal, sphenoid and ethnoid bones, which join the nasal cavity through small orifices called ostia. Their function is to warm the air before it reaches the inferior respiratory tract.

choanae
Two large orifices that form the posterior limit of the nasal fossae. They are bordered by the nasal septum, the roof of the mouth and the lateral walls of the nasal fossae, and connect directly with the oral pharynx.

orifices of the Eustachian tube
Two orifices located laterally in the superior pharynx or nasal pharynx which, through ducts, connect with the cavities of the middle ear, allowing air to pass through them.

nasal vestibule
Widenings that constitute the initial part of the two nasal fossae. The vestibule, like the other parts of the upper airway, is covered by a mucosa rich in mucous glands and villi that filter the air.

nasal pharynx
The nasal fossae end at the nasal pharynx which is the upper part of a larger duct called the pharynx, which has both digestive and respiratory functions, although in the nasal pharynx they are mainly respiratory.

oral pharynx
The central portion of the pharynx which is located immediately behind the oral cavity. It has both digestive and respiratory functions, ingesting food and inspiring and expiring air.

nasal orifices
The anterior openings of the nasal fossae which open to the exterior and are located in the inferior part of the nose.

laryngeal pharynx
The lower part of the pharynx, which connects directly with the prolongation of the digestive system (oesophagus) and with the inferior respiratory tract (larynx), sharing functions with both systems.

107

hard palate
The anterior part of the palate, which is supported by the maxilla and is also known as the bony palate.

soft palate
The posterior part of the palate formed of muscle and ligaments. It has no bony support.

adenoid tonsils
Spongy structures located in the posterior wall of the oral pharynx. They are formed of lymphoid tissue and form part of the body's defence system, filtering microscopic impurities and organisms from the inspired air.

lingual tonsils
Structures similar to the palatine tonsils located in the laryngeal pharynx.

palatine tonsils
Two structures whose shape, constitution and function are very similar to those of the adenoid tonsils, and which are located in the lateral walls of the oral pharynx.

▼ FRONTAL VIEW

frontal paranasal sinuses
Two cavities located in the frontal bone which end in the nasal cavity through orifices located behind the conchae called meati.

palate or **roof of the mouth**
A horizontal partition that separates the nasal fossae from the oral cavity. The hard palate is supported by bone, while the soft palate is composed of muscles and ligaments.

nasal septum
A cartilaginous partition covered by a mucous membrane that separates the nasal fossae into two cavities.

maxillary sinus
Two cavities located in the zygomatic bones which connect with the nasal cavity through orifices situated behind the conchae called the meati.

conchae
Bony protuberances covered by nasal mucosa located in the lateral walls of the nasal fossae. There are generally three: the superior, middle and inferior.

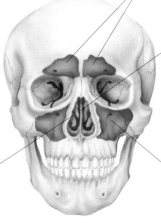

LARYNX AND TRACHEA

▼ ANTERIOR VIEW

▼ INNER VIEW

hyoid bone
A U-shaped bone located in the anterior part of the neck, which serves as the insertion point of the muscles of the tongue, pharynx and larynx.

epiglottis
A cartilaginous structure that acts as a cover for the orifice of entrance to the inferior respiratory tract. When open, it allows air to enter or leave. When shut, it protects the respiratory system from the entrance of food.

glottis
The glottis is the cavity giving entry to the larynx. It is formed of a superior part located over the vocal chords known as the vestibule of the larynx and an inferior portion called the subglottic space.

thyroid cartilage
A cartilaginous structure formed by two lateral laminae that are joined anteriorly, and form the anterior and lateral walls of the larynx. Its anterior border forms a protuberance in the neck, called the Adam's apple, which is more prominent in men.

larynx
A tubular duct located in the anterior part of the neck and formed of cartilaginous structures united by ligaments and muscles. It connects the pharynx and epiglottis with the trachea. The larynx contains a cavity called the glottis and membranous folds known as the vocal cords.

Morgagni's ventricle
A recess in the lateral wall of the larynx into which the laryngeal sacculus opens.

108

cricoid cartilage
A ring-shaped cartilage that surrounds the larynx and is located below the thyroid cartilage.

arytenoid cartilages
Two small, triangular cartilages at the back of the larynx to which the vocal folds are attached.

thyroid cartilage
Two laminae that form the anterior and lateral walls of the larynx, but not its posterior part.

trachea
The inferior prolongation of the larynx, with the same tubular shape. It is formed of a series of cartilaginous rings. Its function is to allow the inspired and expired air to pass.

carina
The area in which the trachea bifurcates into the two main bronchi.

vocal cords
Membranous folds located in the middle zone of the glottis. The upper and lower vocal chords vibrate as air passes, producing sounds that are modulated by the brain to form the words that we speak. Stretching the vocal chords alters the pitch of the voice.

tracheal cartilages
Cartilaginous rings that form the walls of the trachea. They do not form a complete circle, remaining open in the posterior part, where muscular fibres complete the circle, allowing the cartilage to contract or dilate.

tracheal mucosa
A fine mucosa that lines the interior of the trachea. It is rich in glands and covered by fine filaments or cilia that filter the air.

cricoid cartilage
A ring-shaped cartilage that surrounds the larynx and marks the inferior limit between the larynx and the trachea.

right and left main bronchi
The final part of the trachea bifurcates to form two lateral ducts called the right and left main bronchi, which have the same tubular form and cartilaginous structure. After a brief extrapulmonary section, the two bronchi enter the lungs.

LUNGS

segmental bronchi
Within each pulmonary lobe, the bronchi undergo successive ramifications which go to the various segments of the lungs.

lobular bronchi
The lobules are small divisions within each lobar segment which are reached by the intersegmental bronchi.

trachea
The inferior prolongation of the larynx, with the same tubular shape. It is formed of a series of cartilaginous rings. Its function is to allow the inspired and expired air to pass, filtering it through a mucous layer containing prolongations or cilia and secretory mucous glands.

arch of the aorta
The aorta ascends from the heart, and then turns left and descends passing over the left main bronchus. It has arterial branches that go towards the head.

pleura
A double membrane that covers the lungs. The internal layer is attached directly to the pulmonary tissue and is known as the pleural viscera. The external layer, known as the parietal pleura, is attached to the structures surrounding the lungs: the ribs, diaphragm, mediastinum, etc.

main bronchi
The right and left bronchi which, after a short extrapulmonary section, enter the lungs becoming the intrapulmonary main bronchi.

pulmonary parenchyma
The connective tissue that forms the interior of the lungs. It is extremely elastic and surrounds the bronchi, alveoli, blood vessels and nerves.

lobar bronchi
The divisions of the main bronchi within the lungs. They go to each of the pulmonary lobes: superior, middle and inferior in the right lung, and superior and inferior in the left lung.

diaphragm
A flat muscle that separates the thoracic cavity from the abdominal cavity and supports the lungs.

cariodphrenic pleural sinuses
The angles formed between the surfaces of the lungs that meet the heart and the diaphragm.

109

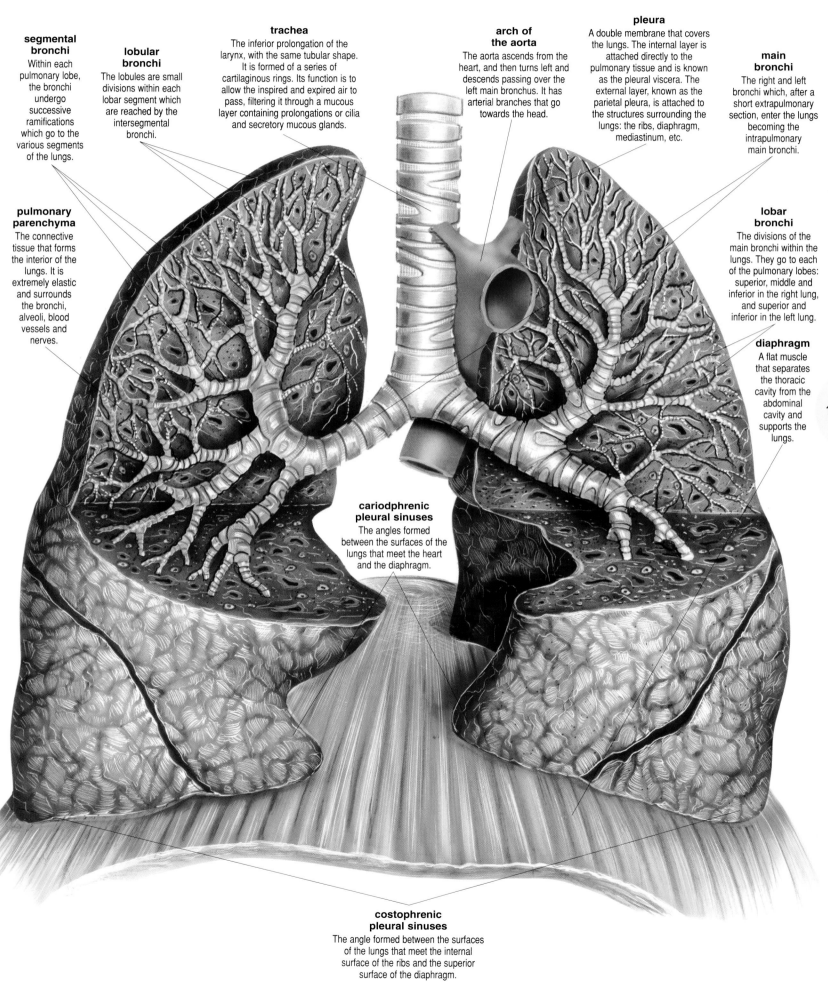

costophrenic pleural sinuses
The angle formed between the surfaces of the lungs that meet the internal surface of the ribs and the superior surface of the diaphragm.

PULMONARY LOBES AND SEGMENTS

RIGHT LUNG

LEFT LUNG

horizontal fissure of the right lung
A sulcus that separates the superior lobe from the middle lobe.

pulmonary hila
Orifices located in the inner faces of both lungs which give entry to the bronchi, the blood vessels and the nerves.

oblique fissure of the left lung
A fissure that separates the superior and inferior lobes of the left lung.

main bronchi
The trachea bifurcates into the two main bronchi which enter the lungs.

pulmonary arteries
The pulmonary artery that carries blood from the right ventricle of the heart to the lungs to exchange the carbon dioxide for oxygen. It divides into the two right and left pulmonary arteries and is the only artery that transports deoxygenated blood.

pulmonary veins
The two right and two left right pulmonary veins carry the oxygenated blood to the left atrium of the heart, from where it passes to the left ventricle and is distributed throughout the body.

110

oblique fissure of the right lung
A sulcus that separates the middle lobe from the inferior lobe of the lung.

BRONCHO-PULMONARY SEGMENTS

RIGHT LUNG

LEFT LUNG

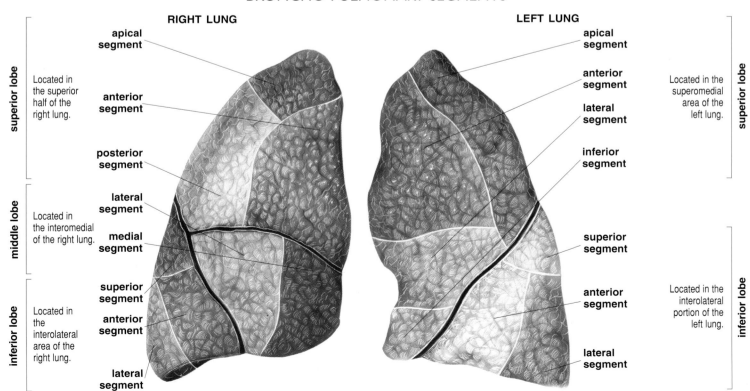

superior lobe
Located in the superior half of the right lung.

apical segment

anterior segment

posterior segment

middle lobe
Located in the interomedial of the right lung.

lateral segment

medial segment

inferior lobe
Located in the interolateral area of the right lung.

superior segment

anterior segment

lateral segment

apical segment

anterior segment

lateral segment

inferior segment

superior segment

anterior segment

lateral segment

superior lobe
Located in the superomedial area of the left lung.

inferior lobe
Located in the interolateral portion of the left lung.

BRANCHES OF THE BRONCHIAL TREE

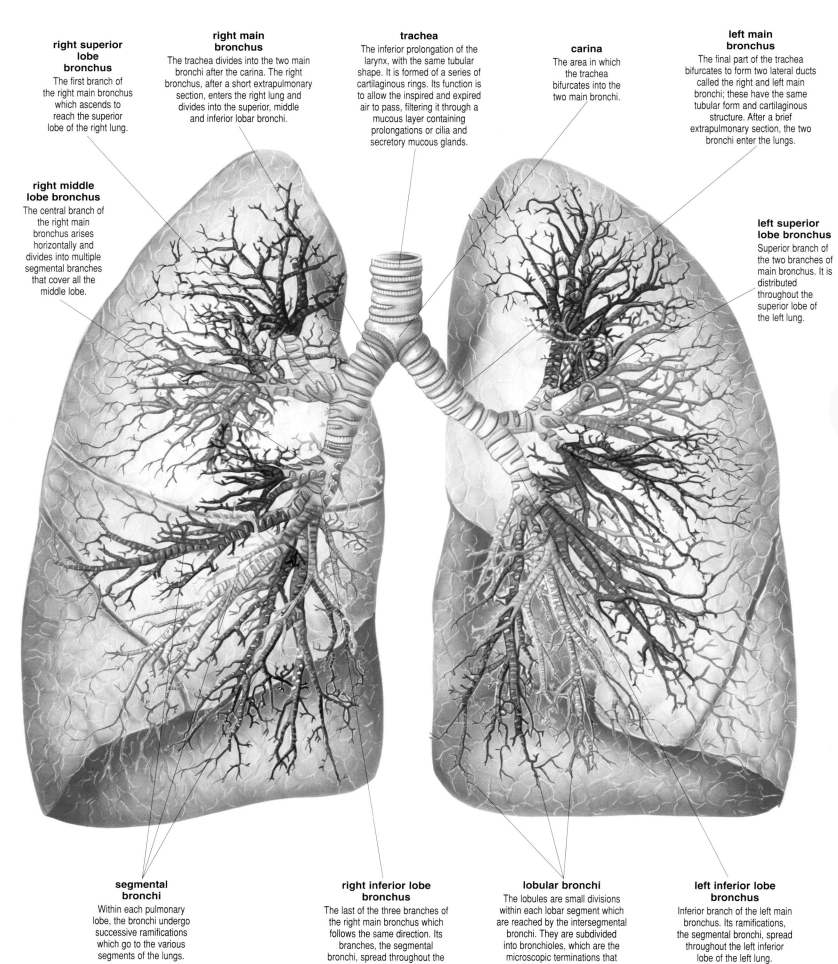

right superior lobe bronchus
The first branch of the right main bronchus which ascends to reach the superior lobe of the right lung.

right main bronchus
The trachea divides into the two main bronchi after the carina. The right bronchus, after a short extrapulmonary section, enters the right lung and divides into the superior, middle and inferior lobar bronchi.

trachea
The inferior prolongation of the larynx, with the same tubular shape. It is formed of a series of cartilaginous rings. Its function is to allow the inspired and expired air to pass, filtering it through a mucous layer containing prolongations or cilia and secretory mucous glands.

carina
The area in which the trachea bifurcates into the two main bronchi.

left main bronchus
The final part of the trachea bifurcates to form two lateral ducts called the right and left main bronchi; these have the same tubular form and cartilaginous structure. After a brief extrapulmonary section, the two bronchi enter the lungs.

right middle lobe bronchus
The central branch of the right main bronchus arises horizontally and divides into multiple segmental branches that cover all the middle lobe.

left superior lobe bronchus
Superior branch of the two branches of main bronchus. It is distributed throughout the superior lobe of the left lung.

111

segmental bronchi
Within each pulmonary lobe, the bronchi undergo successive ramifications which go to the various segments of the lungs.

right inferior lobe bronchus
The last of the three branches of the right main bronchus which follows the same direction. Its branches, the segmental bronchi, spread throughout the inferior lobe of the right lung.

lobular bronchi
The lobules are small divisions within each lobar segment which are reached by the intersegmental bronchi. They are subdivided into bronchioles, which are the microscopic terminations that reach the pulmonary alveoli.

left inferior lobe bronchus
Inferior branch of the left main bronchus. Its ramifications, the segmental bronchi, spread throughout the left inferior lobe of the left lung.

MICROSCOPIC STRUCTURE OF THE LUNGS

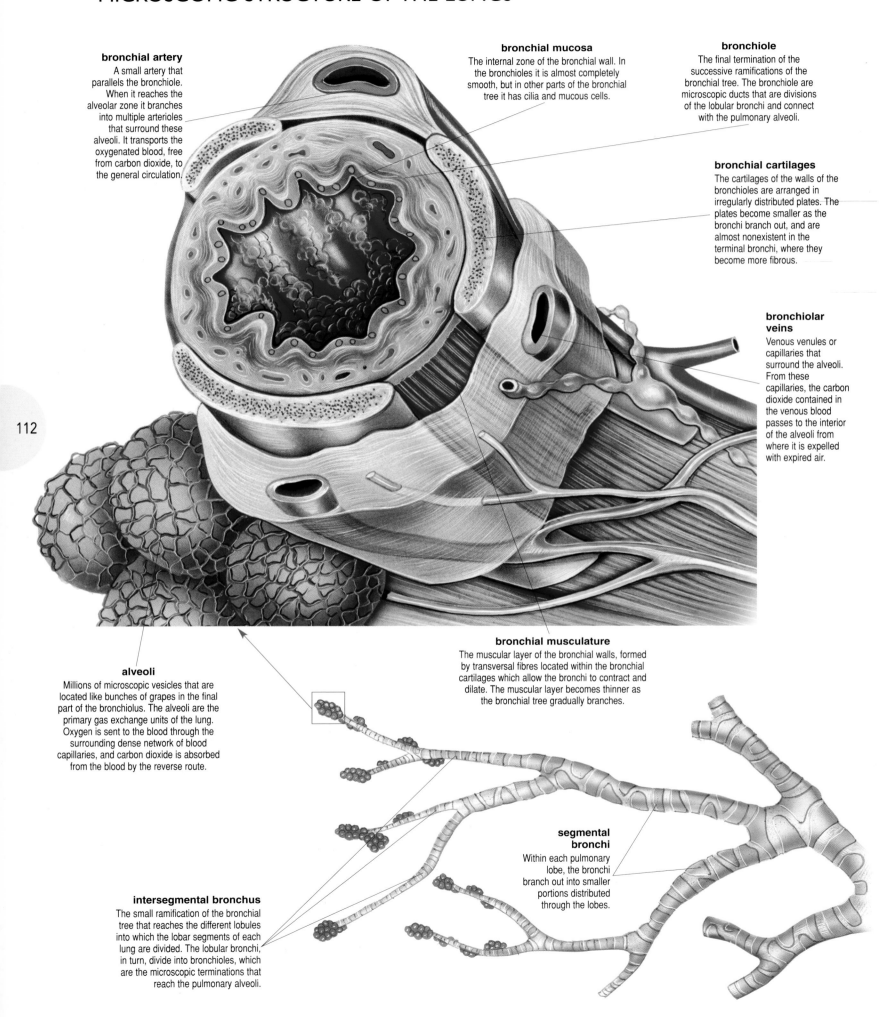

bronchial artery
A small artery that parallels the bronchiole. When it reaches the alveolar zone it branches into multiple arterioles that surround these alveoli. It transports the oxygenated blood, free from carbon dioxide, to the general circulation.

bronchial mucosa
The internal zone of the bronchial wall. In the bronchioles it is almost completely smooth, but in other parts of the bronchial tree it has cilia and mucous cells.

bronchiole
The final termination of the successive ramifications of the bronchial tree. The bronchiole are microscopic ducts that are divisions of the lobular bronchi and connect with the pulmonary alveoli.

bronchial cartilages
The cartilages of the walls of the bronchioles are arranged in irregularly distributed plates. The plates become smaller as the bronchi branch out, and are almost nonexistent in the terminal bronchi, where they become more fibrous.

bronchiolar veins
Venous venules or capillaries that surround the alveoli. From these capillaries, the carbon dioxide contained in the venous blood passes to the interior of the alveoli from where it is expelled with expired air.

112

alveoli
Millions of microscopic vesicles that are located like bunches of grapes in the final part of the bronchiolus. The alveoli are the primary gas exchange units of the lung. Oxygen is sent to the blood through the surrounding dense network of blood capillaries, and carbon dioxide is absorbed from the blood by the reverse route.

bronchial musculature
The muscular layer of the bronchial walls, formed by transversal fibres located within the bronchial cartilages which allow the bronchi to contract and dilate. The muscular layer becomes thinner as the bronchial tree gradually branches.

segmental bronchi
Within each pulmonary lobe, the bronchi branch out into smaller portions distributed through the lobes.

intersegmental bronchus
The small ramification of the bronchial tree that reaches the different lobules into which the lobar segments of each lung are divided. The lobular bronchi, in turn, divide into bronchioles, which are the microscopic terminations that reach the pulmonary alveoli.

THE MEDIASTINUM

THE MEDIASTINUM

The middle region of the thorax, limited laterally by the lungs, posteriorly by the vertebral column and anteriorly by the sternum. The mediastinum contains the thymus, heart, the thoracic aorta and its branches, the inferior vena cava, the trachea and main bronchi and the oesophagus. The portion located in front of the trachea is called the anterior mediastinum, and the portion behind the trachea the posterior mediastinum.

pleura
A double membrane that covers the lungs. The internal layer is attached directly to the pulmonary tissue and is known as the pleural viscera. The external layer, known as the parietal pleura, is attached to the structures surrounding the lungs: the ribs, diaphragm, mediastinum, etc.

oesophagus
A cylindrical duct that descends the thoracic cavity, connecting the pharynx with the stomach.

bifurcation of the trachea
The trachea terminates in a bifurcation which divides it into the right and left main bronchi which enter the respective lungs.

left subclavian artery
An artery that originates in the arch of the aorta and ascends to the upper limbs which it supplies with arterial blood.

right pulmonary artery
The pulmonary artery that carries blood from the right ventricle of the heart to the lungs to exchange the carbon dioxide for oxygen. It divides into the right and left pulmonary arteries and is the only artery that transports deoxygenated blood.

right inferior lobar bronchus
The main bronchi divide into the lobar bronchi when they enter the lungs. There are three lobar bronchi in the right lung and two in the left lung, which go to the respective lobules.

left pulmonary veins
The two left and two right pulmonary veins carry the oxygenated blood to the left atrium of the heart, from where it passes to the left ventricle and is distributed throughout the body.

horizontal fissure
A sulcus that separates the superior and middle lobes of the right lung.

left pulmonary artery
The pulmonary artery or trunk carries blood from the right ventricle of the heart to the lungs to exchange the carbon dioxide for oxygen. It divides into the right and left pulmonary arteries.

oblique fissure of the right lung
The right lung is divided in three lobes: superior, middle and inferior, separated by fissures. The oblique fissure separates the middle lobe from the inferior lobe.

left atrium
The blood oxygenated in the lungs is transported by the pulmonary veins to the left atrium and from there to the left ventricle.

pleural cavity
The space between the visceral pleura and the parietal pleura. Under normal conditions it is a virtual cavity, because the two walls are united.

pericardium
A layer of fibrous tissue that encloses the walls of the heart. Like the pleura, it consists of the internal or visceral wall and the external or parietal wall.

costophrenic pleural sinuses
The angle formed between the surfaces of the lungs that meet the internal face of the ribs and the superior face of the diaphragm.

oblique fissure of the left lung
A fissure that separates the superior and inferior lobes of the left lung.

diaphragm
A flat muscle that separates the thoracic and abdominal cavities and supports the lungs.

liver
A large organ located under the right lung from which it is separated by the diaphragm. Its left portions extends below the heart.

inferior vena cava
A large blood vessel that collects the venous blood from the inferior part of the body and transports it to the right atrium. In the subdiaphragmatic region it receives the hepatic veins.

right pulmonary veins
The right pulmonary veins carry the oxygenated blood from the right lung to the left atrium of the heart. Each lung has two pulmonary veins.

aorta
The aorta originates in the heart and crosses the mediastinum vertically. When it passes through the diaphragm it becomes the abdominal aorta.

stomach
A large saccular organ that receives food from the oesophagus and stores it during the digestive process. The walls of the stomach contain glands that secrete gastric juices that help break down the food. The contraction of the stomach walls mixes the food within to aid digestion.

wall of the left ventricle
The left ventricle of the heart receives the oxygenated blood coming from the left atrium and expels it to the aorta and thus the whole body by contractions of the powerful musculature of its walls.

113

THE URINARY SYSTEM

▼ FRONTAL GENERAL VIEW (MALE)

inferior vena cava
A thick vein that ascends the abdomen. It collects the venous blood from the abdominal organs and carries it to the heart.

renal hilum
A fissure in the internal part of the kidneys through which the renal blood vessels and the ureters, ducts that transport the urine, enter and leave the kidneys.

renal pelvis
A large cavity that collects the urine from the renal hilus. It narrows to form the ureter.

ureters
Two irregularly shaped ducts that descend from the renal pelvises, crossing the posterior part of the abdominal cavity vertically. They carry the urine to the bladder to be expelled.

trigone of the bladder
A triangular formation located in the internal surface of the posterior wall of the bladder. The posterior points are the ureteric orifices, which are joined by a muscular rim, and the anterior point is the neck of the bladder.

prostate
A glandular organ, found only in men, which is attached to the inferior part of the bladder, surrounding the opening of the urethra. Its glands produce secretions that help to form the semen.

suprarenal capsules
Structures located over the kidneys which house the suprarenal glands.

kidneys
Two organs located in the abdominal cavity, behind the peritoneum. The kidneys filter and cleanse the blood and also create the urine from the body's waste products.

renal artery
The right and left renal arteries are branches of the aorta which enter the kidneys through the renal hilus.

renal veins
The right and left renal veins carry filtered blood from the kidney to the inferior vena cava.

abdominal aorta
The portion of the aorta that crosses the abdomen and takes the arterial blood from the heart to the various abdominal organs.

bladder
A hollow organ located in the middle inferior area of the pelvic cavity, which receives the ureters. The walls are formed of musculomembranous tissue and its function is to retain the urine until it is expelled.

orifices of the ureter
Orifices that allow the urine to pass from the ureter to the bladder.

neck of the bladder
Located at the base of the bladder where the urethra begins, the sphincters of the neck of the bladder control urination.

masculine urethra
A duct that carries the urine from the urinary bladder to be expelled during urination. It is longer than the female urethra as it must descend the penis. It is divided into three parts: the prostate urethra, the membranous urethra and the penile urethra.

glans
Enlarged final part of the penis, which is covered by a fold of skin called the prepuce.

external urethral orifice or meatus
The point where urine is expelled from the urethra.

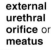

external urethral orifice or meatus
The orifice where the urine from the female urethra is expelled.

female urethra
A duct that connects the female bladder with the exterior.

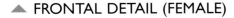

▲ FRONTAL DETAIL (FEMALE)

114

KIDNEYS

▼ EXTERNAL VIEW

KIDNEYS

Two organs located in the abdominal cavity, behind the peritoneum. The kidneys filter and cleanse the blood and also create urine from the body's waste products. The kidneys are shaped like beans and have an interior concavity that contains the renal hilus.

suprarenal capsule
A structure located on the superior pole of each kidney. It contains the suprarenal glands that secrete hormones such as adrenalin, noradrenaline, glucocorticoids, mineralocorticoids and some sexual hormones.

renal hilum
A fissure in the internal part of the kidneys through which the renal blood vessels and the ureters, ducts that transport the urine, enter and leave the kidneys.

renal artery
A branch of the abdominal aorta that enters the kidney through the renal hilum. Within the kidney it branches into multiple arterioles that carry the blood to the functional units of the kidney, the nephrons, where the blood is purified.

ureter
An irregularly shaped duct that descends from the renal pelvis, crossing the posterior part of the abdominal cavity vertically. It carries urine to the urinary bladder to be expelled.

renal vein
A vein that leaves the kidney through the renal hilum and terminates in the inferior vena cava. It originates in the interior of the kidney through the union of multiple venules that come from the renal functional units, the nephrons, and which carry the blood purified of waste products.

▼ INTERNAL VIEW

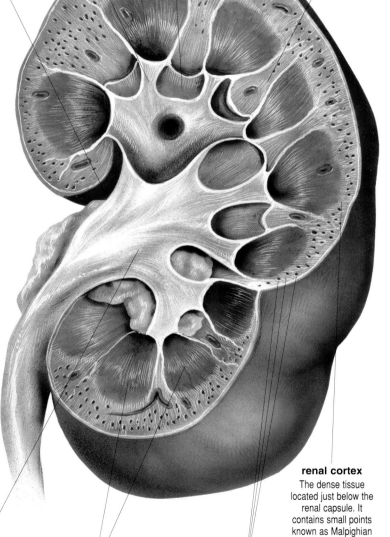

renal papilla
The renal papillae are the internal vertices of Malpighian pyramids, through which the urine is transported to the minor chalices.

renal sinus
A cavity located in the centre of the kidney, surrounded by the renal marrow. It contains the renal calyces and the renal pelvis.

renal calyx
The renal calyces are chambers composed of many smaller or minor calices that receive the urine from the thousands of tiny renal papillae. Each kidney has three major calyces, the superior, medial and inferior.

renal capsule
A fibrous membrane that covers all the external surface of the kidney except for an orifice in the internal face called the renal hilum.

renal marrow
The layer lying just below the renal cortex, which contains the conical structures known as Malpighian pyramids.

renal cortex
The dense tissue located just below the renal capsule. It contains small points known as Malpighian corpuscles.

renal pelvis
The renal pelvis is a basin at the base of the kidney which collects urine from the renal calyces and carries it to the ureter.

Malpighian pyramids
Conical formations consisting of multiple ducts that filter and purify the blood and also manufacture and transport the urine with waste products.

Malpighian corpuscles
Small structures located in the renal cortex that constitute the fundamental part of the functional units of the kidney, the nephrons, where the blood is filtered.

MICROSCOPIC STRUCTURE OF THE KIDNEY

**afferent
arteriole**
A small artery
that carries blood
to the Malpighian
corpuscle for
filtration. The
arterioles are the
continuation of the
branches of the
renal artery.

**glomerular basal
membrane**
A porous membrane that
lines the tiny blood vessels
composing the renal
glomerulus which are
essential for the complicated
process of glomerular
filtration of the blood.

**Bowman's
capsule**
An external membranous
layer that covers the
renal glomerulus.

NEPHRON
The functional unit of the kidney, which may contain a
million or more. It consists of two well defined parts: the
Malpighian corpuscle and a tubular system made up
of the proximal contouring tubules, Henle's loop
and the distal contouring tubules. Blood is filtered
in the nephron to remove impurities and waste
products, which are expelled in the urine.

RENAL GLOMERULUS

**distal
convoluting
tubule**
A tubular system
which is a
continuation of
Henle's loop and
which returns to the
area of Malpighian
corpuscle.

**proximal
convoluting
tubule**
The first part of the
tubular system through
which the product of
the filtration of the
blood leaves. It is
located near to
Malpighian corpuscle.

**Malpighian
corpuscle**

116

**collecting
tubule**
A tubular duct that
receives the distal
convoluting tubules
and collects the
urine, the end
product of renal
filtration. This duct
crosses the renal
marrow and
terminates in the
renal calyces through
the papillae.

**efferent
arteriole**
A small artery that
leaves the Malpighian
corpuscle carrying the
filtered blood. The
efferent arterioles
unite to form the
venules that terminate
in the renal vein.

**juxtaglomerular
apparatus**
A complex structure
located between the
afferent and afferent
arterioles, which
secretes renin, a
substance governing
the operation of the
kidney and acts as
a regulator of blood
pressure.

renal glomerulus
A capillary bed formed
of a compact bunch of
interconnected capillaries,
which constitutes the central
part of the renal corpuscle or
Malpighian corpuscle. Blood
arrives at the glomerulus to
be filtered by the basal
membrane, retaining
proteins, blood globules
and other substances which
can be used by the body
(glomerular filtration).

**Malpighian
corpuscle**
A structure located in the
renal cortex. It receives
afferent arterioles carrying
blood to be filtered and
gives off the efferent
arterioles containing filtered
blood. It contains a great
amount of tiny blood
vessels crowded together
(renal glomerulus),
surrounded by a membrane
(Bowman's capsule).

renal papillae
Orifices through
which the urine
arrives from the
collecting tubules to
the renal calyces.

Henle's loop
A straight, tubular
structure that is a
continuation of the
proximal
convoluting tubule.
It consists of a
descending part
that enters the renal
marrow, and an
ascending part that
returns to the renal
cortex. Its function
is to select the
products obtained
through glomerular
filtration.

THE BLADDER AND URETHRA

▼ INTERNAL VIEW

ureters
Ducts that carry
urine from the kidneys
to the urinary bladder.

ovary
Two female sexual
glands that are
located on either
side of the body
near the ureters.

deferent duct
The excretory duct of
the testis which joins
the excretory duct of the
seminal vesicle to form
the ejaculatory duct.

peritoneum
A serous layer
located above the
bladder that covers
the abdominal cavity.

bladder
A hollow organ that receives
the urine from the ureters. The
bladder walls are formed of
musculomembranous tissue.
The function of the bladders
is to retain the urine until
expulsion.

trigone of the bladder
A triangular area located in
the internal surface of the
posterior wall of the bladder.
The posterior points are the
ureteric orifices, which are
joined by a muscular
rim, and the anterior point is
the neck of the bladder.

neck of the bladder
The area of the floor of the
bladder where the urethra
begins. The muscular
layer of the bladder wall
thickens to form the
internal urethral sphincter.

ureteral meatus
Orifices through which the urine
enters the bladder from the
ureters. The muscular walls of
the bladder form a valve that
prevents a reflux of the urine.

feminine urethra
The female urethra is
much shorter than the
male one, running
from the neck of the
bladder to the urethral
meatus in the vulva.

prostate
A gland found only in males,
which manufactures some
components of the seminal fluid.

prostate urethra
First portion of the masculine
urethra located at the level of
the prostate gland.

membranous urethra
The second part of the masculine
urethra which corresponds to the short
portion that crosses the perineum.

penile urethra
The final part of the male
urethra which runs down the
penis and expels the urine.

labia minora
One of the two mucocutaneous
folds that border the vaginal
orifice laterally.

labia majora
One of the two cutaneous
folds that surround
the smaller lips.

scrotum
A cutaneous
sac located in
the anterior part
of the male
perineum which
contains the
testicles.

glans
The final,
enlarged part
of the penis,
covered by a
retractable layer
of skin known
as the prepuce.

penis
A cylindrical organ located
anterior to the scrotum. It
contains the penile urethra
which expels the urine.

urethral meatus
The external part of
the urethra, through
which urine is expelled.

FEMALE

MALE

117

MALE REPRODUCTIVE SYSTEM

▼ GENERAL VIEW. LATERAL CROSS SECTION

peritoneum
A membrane that lines the abdominal cavity and covers the superior part of the bladder and a substantial part of the anterior face of the rectum.

rectouterine pouch or pouch of Douglas
A fold of the peritoneum that forms a cul-de-sac between the bladder and the rectum.

rectum
The final part of the large intestine. It is located behind the prostate, which may become enlarged enough to be felt by rectal examination.

anus
The external orifice of the large intestine.

prostate
A gland located below the bladder. Its function is to produce a series of secretions that are mixed with sperm in the urethra to form the seminal fluid that is expelled by ejaculation.

perineum
A region that extends from the posterior part of the scrotal sac to the anus.

sigmoid colon
The final part of the descending colon that ends at the rectum.

urinary bladder
A saccular organ forming part of the urinary system in which the urine is stored before being expelled. It is located above the prostate.

ureter
A duct that connects the kidney with the bladder.

iliac veins and arteries
The iliac veins and arteries have branches that supply and drain blood from the reproductive apparatus.

symphysis of the pubis
A joint formed by the union of the pubic bones which constitutes the anterior limit of the pelvic cavity.

cavernous bodies of the penis
Cylinders with a spongy structure located in the dorsal part of the penis. They fill with blood during sexual arousal, causing the penis to become enlarged and erect.

urethra
A duct that carries urine from the urinary bladder down the penis to be expelled, and semen from the deferent ducts which is ejaculated. It consists of three parts: the prostatic, membranous and penile urethra.

penis
The external male genital organ, which enlarges and becomes erect during arousal. It houses the urethra which expels the urine and allows semen to be deposited in the vagina during copulation.

glans
Conical swelling located in the distal end of the penis, from which it is separated by the balanopreputial sulcus.

urinary meatus
External orifice of the urethra, located in the vertex of the glans. Through it the semen and urine are expelled.

erectile tissue
The spongy tissue that surrounds the urethra. During sexual arousal it fills with blood causing the penis to enlarge and become erect.

scrotum
A saccular structure located in the anterior zone of the perineum, behind the penis, and hangs between both thighs. It contains the testicles.

testicles
Ovoid organs contained in the scrotum. They produce spermatozoa, the male reproductive cells, and the hormones responsible for of the appearance of the masculine sexual characteristics.

prepuce or foreskin
The skin that covers the distal end of the glans penis. It may retract to leave the glans uncovered.

118

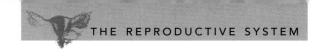
FEMALE REPRODUCTIVE SYSTEM

▼ GENERAL VIEW. LATERAL CROSS-SECTION

ovary
The two ovaries located on each side of the body are the female sexual glands. They have a double function, producing the ova (female sexual cells) and also manufacturing female sexual hormones. This activity begins in puberty and stops at the menopause.

iliac vein and artery
The iliac vein and artery originate in the inferior vena cava and the abdominal aorta respectively and descend to the pelvic area where they ramify into the branches that irrigate and collect blood from the reproductive apparatus.

ureter
A duct that connects the kidney with the urinary bladder. In this area it passes close to the Fallopian tubes and the uterus.

sigmoid colon
The distal part of the descending colon that ends at the rectum.

Fallopian tubes
The two Fallopian tubes join the ovaries to the superior part of the uterine cavity. Their function is to transport the egg to the uterus after it is released by the ovary.

broad ligament
A large ligament that unites the female uterus and other genital organs with the walls of the pelvic cavity.

peritoneum
A membrane that lines the abdominal cavity and covers the superior part of the bladder and a substantial part of the anterior face of the rectum.

rectouterine pouch or **pouch of Douglas**
A fold of the peritoneum that forms a cul-de-sac behind the uterine cavity.

bladder
A saccular organ in which the urine is stored before being expelled.

rectum
The final portion of the digestive system. It is located immediately behind the uterus, whose posterior wall it supports.

uterus
A hollow organ formed of thick muscular walls, located in the medial part of the pelvic cavity and divided into three sections: the wider uterine body, the medial uterine isthmus and the thinner uterine neck. The uterus lodges the fertilized egg as it grows.

symphysis of the pubis
A joint formed by the union of the pubic bones which constitutes the anterior limit of the pelvic cavity.

mount of Venus or **pubis**
A projection in the skin located just under the skin in the superior part of the vulva.

urethral orifice
A small orifice located below the clitoris and above the vaginal orifice through which urine is expelled from the urethra.

clitoris
An erectile organ located in the vertex of union of the labia majora, covered partially by a cutaneous fold.

labia majora
One of the two cutaneous folds that surround the labia minora.

labia minora
One of the two mucocutaneous folds that border the vaginal orifice laterally.

vaginal orifice
The external orifice of the vagina, which is covered by a fine membrane called the hymen which is broken when sexual relations are initiated.

vulva
The external female genital organs.

anus
The external orifice of the large intestine.

perineum
A region that extends from the inferior extreme of the vulva to the anus, forming the floor of the pelvic cavity.

vagina
A duct formed of muscle and membrane that originates in the cervical neck and connects with the exterior through the vaginal orifice. Its function is to receive the masculine penis during copulation. It can expand enormously to accommodate the foetus during childbirth.

119

THE PENIS

▼ ANTERIOR VIEW

base of the penis
Also called the root of the penis. The area where the penile shaft unites with the inferior part of the abdomen.

penile shaft
The central, cylindrical part of the penis.

glans
A conical swelling located in the distal end of the penis. Its widest part is called the corona of the glans. The urethral meatus opens in its distal part.

scrotum or **scrotal sac**
A saccular structure located in the anterior zone of the perineum, behind the penis, and hanging between both thighs.

pubic hair
Thick, curly hair that covers the inferior part of the abdomen above the penis.

PENIS
The external male genital organ, that enlarges and becomes erect during arousal. It houses the urethra which expels the urine and allows semen to be deposited in the vagina during copulation. It consists of the base, the shaft and the distal extreme or glans.

prepuce or foreskin
The skin that covers the glans. It may retract to leave the glans uncovered.

balanopreputial sulcus
The sulcus that delimits the crown of the glans and separates it from the penile shaft.

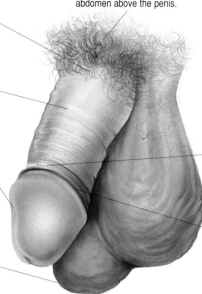

▼ POSTERIOR VIEW

coronal sulcus
A sulcus that crosses the surface of the glans from the urethral meatus to the frenulum. It is uniformly smooth and uniform except in the anterior face.

urethral meatus
The external orifice of the urethra located in the vertex of the glans. Its functions are to expel urine and ejaculate semen.

glans
Conical swelling located in the distal end of the penis from which it is separated by the balanopreputial sulcus.

frenulum
A cutaneous fold that unites the prepuce and the glans in the posterior face of the penis.

penile shaft
The central, cylindrical part of the penis.

prepuce
The skin that covers the distal end of the glans penis. It may retract to leave the glans uncovered.

VULVA

▼ FRONTAL VIEW

mount of Venus or **pubis**
An area located in the superior part of the vulva. From puberty it is covered by thick, heavy pubic hair.

clitoris
An erectile organ located in the vertex of the union of the two labia minora. It is formed of erectile tissue that fills with blood during sexual stimulation.

frenulum of the clitoris
Cutaneous folds of the labia minora in its anterior part which unite in the anterior part of the clitoris in a way that imitates the male frenulum.

urethral orifice
A small orifice located below the clitoris and above the vaginal orifice through which urine is expelled from the urethra.

opening of Bartholin's glands
A pair of glands located between the vagina and the vulva that produce lubrication when stimulated, thus facilitating sexual intercourse. They are also called the greater vestibular glands.

vaginal orifice
The external orifice of the vagina, which is covered by a fine membrane called the hymen which is broken when sexual relations are initiated.

posterior commissure or **fourchette of the vulva**
The angle formed by the union of the posterior parts of the labia majora.

VULVA
The external female genital organs. Located in the inferior zone of the abdomen between the thighs, it constitutes the visible, exterior part of the female reproductive apparatus.

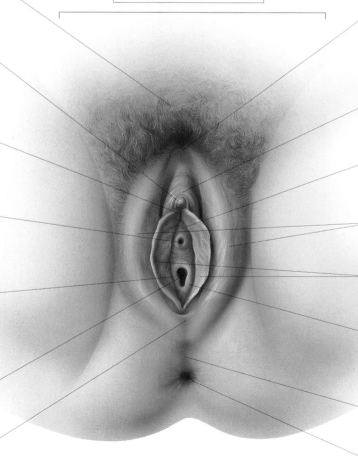

anterior commissure of the labia majora
The angle formed by the union of the posterior parts of the labia majora.

prepuce of the clitoris
A cutaneous fold formed by the anterior part of the labia minora, that covers the clitoris in a similar way to the male prepuce.

vestibule
The vestibule of the vagina is the name given to the cleft or space which is surrounded by the labia minora.

labia majora
One of the two cutaneous folds that surround the labia minora. Their anterior areas are a rosy colour and the posterior areas are somewhat darker.

labia minora
One of the two mucocutaneous folds that border the vaginal orifice laterally.

hymen
An incomplete membrane that partially blocks the vaginal orifice, and is usually broken when sexual relations are initiated. It can adopt very different forms.

perineum
An area located between the thighs that extends from the posterior commissure to the anus.

anus
The external orifice of the rectum and the posterior limit of the perineum.

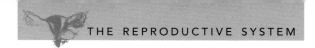

OVARIES, TUBES AND UTERUS

▼ EXTERNAL AND INTERNAL ANTERIOR VIEW

Fallopian tube or uterine tube
The Fallopian tubes are the ducts that connect the ovaries with the uterus. Their function is to collect the ovum, once released from the ovary, and transport it to the uterus. They consist of three portions: the isthmus, the ampulla and the infundibulum. Their walls are formed by an external serous tunica, two medial layers of smooth musculature and one internal mucous layer.

uterus
In the pre-pregnant state, the uterus is the shape and size of a small pear, and is about one inch thick. It contains the fertilized ovum.

mesosalpinx of the broad ligament
A membrane that unites the Fallopian tube with the uterus, ensuring they do not become separated and no released ovum is lost.

cervical neck
The lowest, narrowest part of the uterus, which ends at the vagina.

body of the uterus
The superior, wider part of the uterus which houses the uterine cavity.

endometrium
A membranous lamina that lines the uterine cavity. It holds the fertilized egg and is shed during the menstrual cycle when the women is not pregnant.

myometrium
Three thick layers of smooth muscle that form the greatest part of the uterine walls.

isthmus
A transitional area that unites the body of the uterus with the neck.

uterine ostium
The orifice located in the superior angle of the uterus which connects it to the uterine or Fallopian tube.

isthmus
The narrower middle part of the Fallopian tube that joins the uterine wall.

ampulla
The mid-region of the Fallopian tube. It has thin walls and virtually no muscle.

infundibulum and folds of the uterine tube
The external part of the uterine tube which ends in the fimbriae. It is joined to the ovary by the membranes of the broad ligament. Its function is to capture the ova released by the ovary.

121

ligament of the ovary
The ligament that fixes the internal portion of the ovaries with the superior angles of the uterus.

external cervical orifice
The portion of the cervical neck that connects directly with the vaginal cavity.

ovary
The ovaries are two pink, ovoid glands located on both sides the female pelvic cavity. They are the feminine sexual glands and their activity begins in puberty and stops at the menopause. They produce the ova which are the female sexual cells and the female sexual hormones.

vaginal fornix
The anterior and posterior recesses into which the upper vagina is divided and which are formed by the protrusion of the cervix into the vagina.

transversal mucous folds
A series of circular sulci that cross the internal face of the vaginal mucosa. They correspond to the marks left by the circular muscular fibres.

mucosa layer of the vagina
A fine membrane that lines the surface of the vagina. It is a continuation of the mucosa of the uterus.

vagina
A duct formed of muscle and membrane that originates in the cervical neck and connects with the exterior through the vaginal orifice. Its function is to receive the masculine penis during copulation. It can expand enormously to accommodate the foetus during childbirth.

tunica muscularis of the vagina
The vaginal walls are equipped with two layers of smooth muscular fibres, one longitudinal and the other circular.

round ligament
A cord that unites the wall of the uterine body with the anterior wall of the abdomen, passing through the inguinal canal.

mesometrium of broad ligament
Prolongation of the peritoneal layer that separates the pelvic and abdominal cavities. It is arranged in front, above and behind the uterus and covers the tubes and the ovaries.

transverse muscle of the vagina
A branch of the deep transverse muscle that goes from the cervical neck to the ramus of the ischium.

tunica serosa of the vagina
A thin layer of connective tissue that covers the vaginal walls.

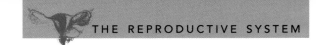

THE BREASTS

breasts
Two hemispheric structures that contain the female mammary glands and are located in the anterosuperior zone of the female chest. Their function is to secrete the breast milk that nourishes the newborn baby.

mammary areola
An area of darker, furrowed skin located around the nipple.

nipple
A protuberance or papilla located in the centre of the mammary areola, which serves as the external orifice for the ducts that carry the breast milk.

Morgagni's tubercules
Small protuberances that cover the mammary areola, giving it a rough, granular aspect. Each contains a sebaceous gland which may contain a hair.

submammary fold
A semicircular crease that lies under each breast where it joins the thorax.

122

▲ LATERAL VIEW OF THE RIGHT BREAST   ▲ FRONTAL VIEW OF THE RIGHT BREAST

MAMMARY GLAND
A lobular, glandular system that produces milky secretions after childbirth and transports them to the nipple by a series of canaliculi.

subcutaneous adipose layer
Abundant adipose or fat tissue located below the skin of the mammary area, which it surrounds and protects.

greater pectoral muscle
Muscle that covers the superoanterior area of the thorax underneath the breast.

gland lobule
The mammary gland is divided into multiple lobules that constitute the functional units.

suspensory ligaments or **ligaments of Cooper**
Located in the posterior face of the mammary gland, the suspensory ligaments unite the breast to the aponeurosis of the greater pectoral muscle located behind it.

lactiferous sinus
Small dilations located in the final part of each of the lactiferous ducts.

lactiferous ducts
Winding ducts that connect each of the gland lobules with the exterior through the nipple, carrying the breast milk.

ribs
Saggital section of the ribs that support the superior pectoral muscle and the breast.

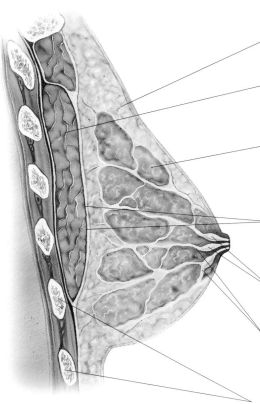

▲ SECTIONS OF THE MAMMARY GLAND

ABDOMEN OF A PREGNANT WOMAN

▼ LATERAL CROSS-SECTION

stomach
The compression suffered by the stomach and the intestinal loops during the last months of pregnancy causes frequent regurgitations which may cause some discomfort such as heartburn or nausea.

liver
During pregnancy the liver is compressed by the enlarged uterus, which may result in difficulties in draining the gallbladder to the intestine.

foetus
The foetus grows from an embryo to the moment of birth. During the later stages of pregnancy, the foetus is perfectly formed.

vertebral column
The increase in abdominal volume during pregnancy moves the centre of gravity forwards, creating a greater anterior curvature of the vertebral column or lordosis, which causes backaches.

intestinal loops of the small intestine
These are also compressed by the increased size of the uterus.

uterus
A hollow cavity with thick muscular walls that progressively expands during pregnancy to accommodate the growing foetus, which occupies nearly all the abdominal cavity of the pregnant woman.

rectum
The final part of the digestive system that communicates with the exterior through the anus. The lack of intestinal mobility due to the pressure of the uterus leads to constipation in some pregnant women.

breasts
During pregnancy, the breasts increase progressively in size and the pigmentation of the areola and the nipple darkens.

vagina
A duct formed of muscle and membrane that originates in the cervical neck and communicates with the exterior through the vaginal orifice. It can expand enormously to accommodate the foetus during childbirth.

cervical neck
The cervical neck remains firmly closed during pregnancy and only becomes dilated in the moments preceding childbirth, in order to allow the passage of the foetus towards the exterior.

bladder
A cavity in which the urine is stored before being expelled. In the final phase of pregnancy, the pressure exerted by the head of the foetus on the bladder causes frequent urination accompanied with discomfort.

placenta
A structure that forms at the end of the first month of pregnancy. It is rich in blood vessels that are attached to the uterine wall and to the foetus by the umbilical cord. It supplies blood and nutrition to the foetus throughout gestation.

umbilical cord
A tubular cord of variable length which unites the centre of the placenta with the foetus. It contains two arteries and a vein which carry arterial blood to and venous blood from the foetus.

umbilical herniation
The intra-abdominal pressure caused by the increased size of the uterus, causes, in many women, a swelling of the umbilicus, which is, in fact, an abdominal hernia through the umbilicus.

amniotic sac
From the beginning of the pregnancy, a membrane forms around the embryo in the shape of a sac which surrounds the foetus during gestation. The sac contains amniotic fluid and only breaks at the moment of birth.

amniotic fluid
A fluid contained inside the amniotic sac, where the foetus is located. It is composed mainly of water, but also contains epithelial cells, foetal urine, salts, enzymes, etc. Its function is to protect the foetus.

symphysis of the pubis
The articulation of the two pubic bones in the anterior part of the pelvis, which, during the final phase of pregnancy and in childbirth, allows a small widening of the channel through which the foetus passes.

123

COMPONENTS OF THE BLOOD

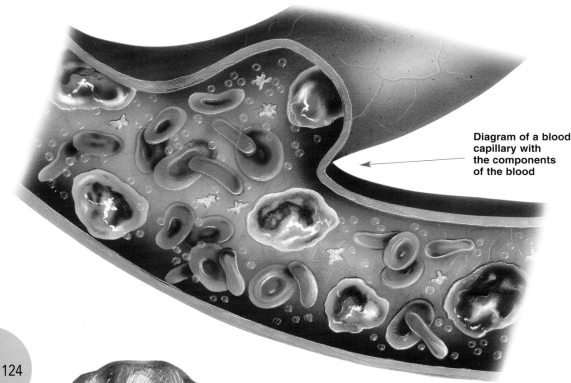

Diagram of a blood capillary with the components of the blood

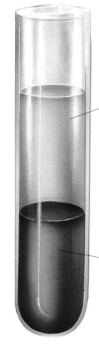

blood plasma
The fluid component fluid of the blood, representing 55–60 per cent of its total volume. Plasma has a yellowish colour and is composed mainly of water, but contains numerous substances, such as proteins, minerals, sugars, enzymes, vitamins, etc.

cellular elements of the blood
The blood cells represent 40–45 per cent of the blood volume and are of three types: red blood cells or erythrocytes, white blood cells or leukocytes, and platelets or thrombocytes.

124

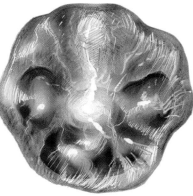

monocyte
A large, bluish blood cell, whose primary function is to defend the body against prolonged or chronic infections.

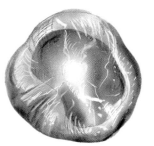

lymphocyte
A bluish cell with a single, large nucleus. There are two types of lymphocytes: T cells which defend the body against viruses and provoke some allergic reactions; and B cells which create antibodies and synthesize some proteins of the immune system.

platelets
Tiny blood cells that, like the red blood cells, have no nucleus. Their main function is to promote the coagulation of the blood to prevent blood loss through haemorrhages and thus maintain haemostasis.

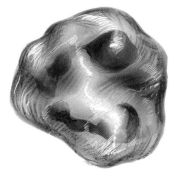

neutrophil
A leukocyte contains several nuclei. Its cytoplasm contains granules that give the cell a violet colour. Neutrophils destroy bacteria by a process known as phagocytosis.

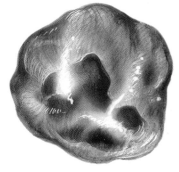

basophil
A leukocyte with several nuclei which contains granules in its cytoplasm that give it a purplish colour. It is part of the body's defence system.

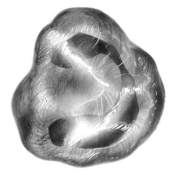

eosinophil
One of the leukocytes that, together with neutrophils and basophils, are called granulocytes. Leukocytes have several nuclei and their cytoplasm is a yellowish-red colour. Their function is to defend the body by blocking the antigen-antibody complexes that form when foreign bodies penetrate the human organism.

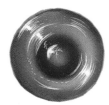

red blood cells
Rounded blood cells with no nucleus which can change shape to adapt to narrow blood capillaries. Blood can contain more than 5 million per mm^2. They contain hemoglobin, which transports oxygen to the cells.

white blood cells
Blood cells, unlike the red cells, etc, have a nucleus. Their main function is to defend the body against the infections caused by foreign germs. Also known as leukocytes, they can cross the pores of the blood vessels to reach any focus of infection. There are several types of white blood cells: granulocytes, lymphocytes and monocytes; granulocytes may be mononuclear or polynuclear (neutrophils, basophils and eosinophils).

SPLEEN

splenic artery
A branch of the celiac trunk which originates in the abdominal aorta and emits arterial branches to the liver, stomach and spleen. The splenic artery emits small branches that supply the pancreas.

splenic vein
A vein formed by the union of several venous branches which leave the spleen. It joins the superior and inferior mesenteric veins to form the portal vein that goes to the liver.

SPLEEN
The spleen is a lymphatic organ located in the superior left quadrant of the abdominal cavity or left hypochondrium, behind the stomach and below the diaphragm. Its function is to destroy the red blood cells after they have completed their mission, and it acts as a reservoir of blood cells and may also produce them. It is also part of the body's immunologic system, contributing to the manufacture of antibodies.

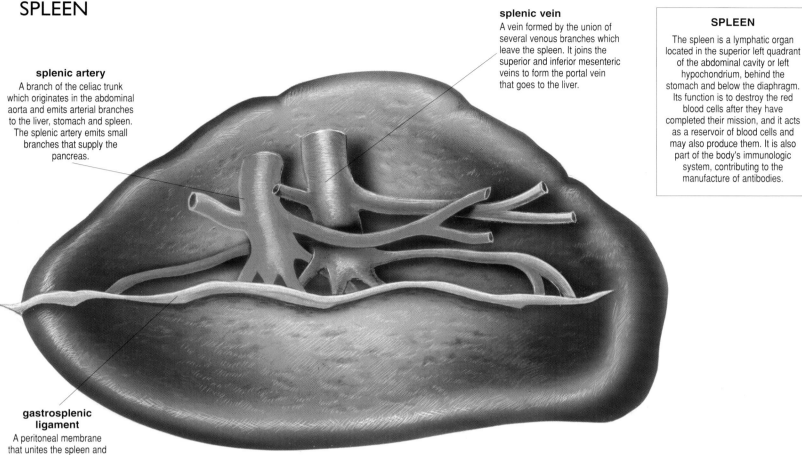

gastrosplenic ligament
A peritoneal membrane that unites the spleen and the greater curvature of the stomach.

125

▲ EXTERNAL VIEW

splenic pulp
The splenic pulp is of two types. The red pulp, which forms 75% of the volume of the spleen, contains massive amounts of red blood cells which give it a deep red colour and the white pulp is formed of lymph tissue. The red pulp contains an intricate arterial network which forms the splenic sinuses.

trabecular arteries and veins
Numerous vascular branches that constitute an intrasplenic network. They ensure that the spleen is supplied with the abundant circulation it needs.

splenic capsule
A cortex formed of membranous connective tissue which covers the spleen. It emits prolongations that divide the organ into lobes or lobules.

hilium of the spleen
A fissure in the internal face of the spleen, which allows the splenic artery and vein to reach the spleen.

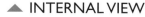 ▲ INTERNAL VIEW

GENERAL VIEW OF THE GLANDULAR SYSTEM

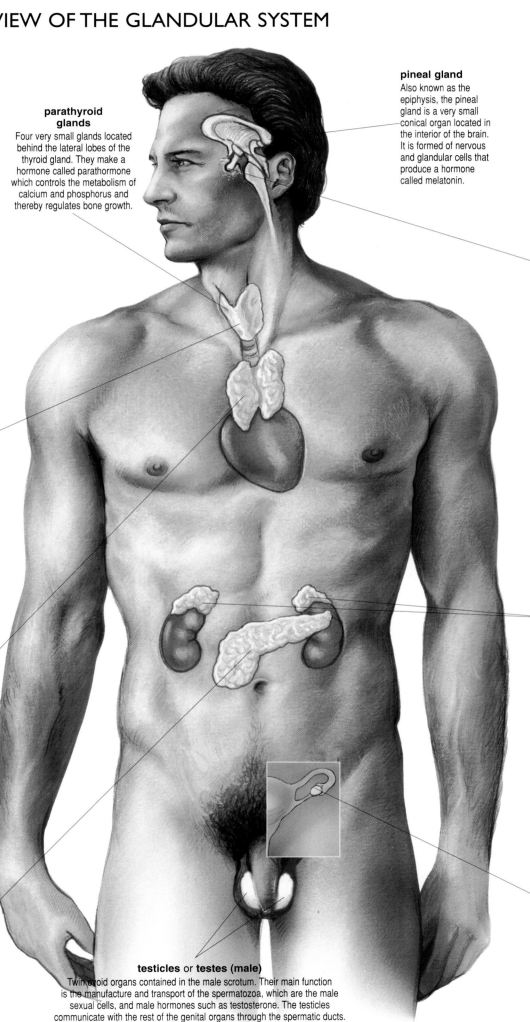

ENDOCRINE SYSTEM

A complex set of interrelated glands that regulate the different metabolic functions of the body and the intensity of the chemical activity of the various cells through the action of substances called hormones. Hormones are chemical substances secreted by a cell or group of cells, which control the function of other cells of the body.

parathyroid glands

Four very small glands located behind the lateral lobes of the thyroid gland. They make a hormone called parathormone which controls the metabolism of calcium and phosphorus and thereby regulates bone growth.

pineal gland

Also known as the epiphysis, the pineal gland is a very small conical organ located in the interior of the brain. It is formed of nervous and glandular cells that produce a hormone called melatonin.

pituitary gland or hypophysis

A small, single ovoid gland located in the interior of the skull within the cavity of the sphenoid bone known as the sella turcica. It is formed of two parts. The anterior or adenohypophysis makes hormones that regulate other glands, such as the thyroid (thyroid stimulating), adrenal cortex (adenocorticotropic) or sexual glands (follicle stimulating and luteinizing), and the hormone that regulates growth. The posterior or neurohypophysis produces hormones that regulate the operation of the kidney (vasopressin) and childbirth and breastfeeding in women (oxytocin).

thyroid

A gland located in the neck, in front of the trachea. It is divided into right and left lobes which are joined by a narrow area called the thyroid isthmus. It produces hormones called thyroxine and triiodothyronine which regulate the basal metabolism and the maturation of the nervous system.

thymus

A gland located in the thoracic cavity, behind the sternum. It consists of right and left lobes and contains lymphoid cells called thymocytes, whose main function is to produce antibodies that defend the body against foreign substances by stimulating the blood lymphocytes. This function is especially important in young children, but seems to be less so in adults.

adrenal or suprarenal glands

Twin glands located at the superior pole of the kidneys. They are formed of two parts, the peripheral or adrenal cortex and the central or adrenal medulla. The adrenal cortex produces mineral-corticoids that maintain the balance between fluids and different minerals of the body, glucocorticoids which regulate the metabolism of glucose, fats and proteins, and small amounts of sexual hormones. The adrenal medulla makes hormones called adrenalin and noradrenaline that act on the nervous system and regulate stress.

ovaries (female)

Twin glands located inside the female pelvic cavity that remain inactive until puberty. Once activated, they have a double function: to manufacture the female sexual cells or ova, that are released in each ovarian cycle; and to manufacture oestrogen and progesterone, the female hormones, which determine the appearance of female characteristics and regulate the menstrual cycle. The ovaries communicate with the rest of the sexual organs through the Fallopian tubes.

pancreas

An organ located in the superior part of the abdominal cavity which has both exocrine and endocrine functions. The exocrine function consists of the secretion of pancreatic fluids to the duodenum to aid the digestion of foods. The endocrine function is the secretion of insulin and glucagon, hormones that enter the blood stream and regulate the uptake of glucose, the main cell nutrient.

testicles or testes (male)

Twin ovoid organs contained in the male scrotum. Their main function is the manufacture and transport of the spermatozoa, which are the male sexual cells, and male hormones such as testosterone. The testicles communicate with the rest of the genital organs through the spermatic ducts.

HYPOPHYSEAL CONTROL

PITUITARY GLAND

Also known as the hypophysis. A small, single ovoid gland, located in the interior of the skull within the cavity of the sphenoid bone known as the sella turcica. In a complex system, governed by a superior structure called the hypothalamus, the pituitary gland regulates the hormonal secretions of the other glands in the body.

neurosecretory cells
The neurosecretory cells are located in the hypothalamus. They secrete hormones called neurosecretory substances, which are carried by the hypothalamus-hypophysial portal system to the adenohypophysis, where they regulate the glandular cells which stimulate the production of hormones. They are called hormone regulation factors.

adenohypophysis
The anterior lobe of the pituitary gland. It contains a series of glandular cells that, when stimulated by the neurosecretory substances produced in the hypothalamus, secrete different types of hormones which stimulate the other glands of the body, such as the thyroid, suprarenal or sexual glands, and others that act on specific tissues, such as the growth hormone.

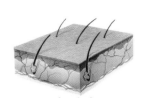

stimulating hormone of the melanocytes
A hormone whose production is governed by the pineal gland. It stimulates the cells of the dermis to produce melanin, the pigment that colours the skin.

hypothalamus
A nervous organ located in the base of the brain, in the floor and lateral walls of the third ventricle. It contains numerous neurological centres that regulate activities such as sight, and sleep and, through nervous stimuli and hormonal secretions, the operation of the hypophysis.

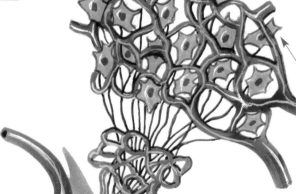

antidiuretic hormone or vasopressin
A hormone produced by the neurohypophysis that regulates the amount of water the kidney reabsorbs, thereby controlling the amount of urine produced.

hypophysial stem
The hypophysis is united to the hypothalamus of the brain through a pedicle or hypophysial stem, which contains some nervous terminations and a dense network of blood vessels that unite both structures.

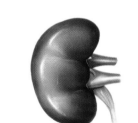

corticotropin
A hormone produced by the adenohypophysis which stimulates the cortex of the suprarenal glands, causing them to secrete glucocorticoids and mineral-corticoids.

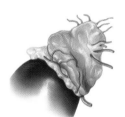

oxytocin
A hormone produced by the neurohypophysis that acts on the uterine musculature, causing the contractions which occur during childbirth, and on the mammary glands, facilitating the production of breast milk.

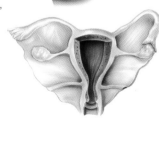

thyrotropin
Adenohypophysial hormone which stimulates the thyroid gland to produce the thyroid hormones, thyroxine and triiodothyronine.

follicle-stimulating hormone
An adenohypophysial hormone that begins to secrete during puberty and acts on the ovaries, stimulating the development of the follicles. In men, it acts on the testicles, initiating the process of production of spermatozoa.

luteinizing hormone
A hormone produced by the adenohypophysis which complements the follicle-stimulating hormone and regulates ovulation in women and the production of testosterone in men.

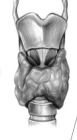

growth hormone
The growth hormone is an adenohypophysial hormone that does not act on another gland, but mainly on growing tissues, where it increases the synthesis of proteins and facilitates the production of energy from fats.

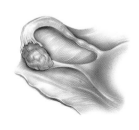

neurohypophysis
The posterior lobe of the hypophysis. It is attached to the hypothalamus by nerve fibres from the nervous centres of the hypothalamus. It produces two types of hormone: the antidiuretic hormone or vasopressin and oxytocin.

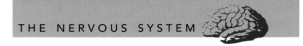

THE NERVOUS SYSTEM

▼ DORSAL GENERAL VIEW

ORGANIZATION OF THE NERVOUS SYSTEM

The nervous system is formed by a set of interconnected organs whose complex operation allows it to control the rest of the body's systems. There is a central nervous system, formed of the brain (cerebrum, mesencephalon, medulla oblongata and cerebellum) and the spinal cord, and a peripheral nervous system, formed of the ganglia and the nerves.

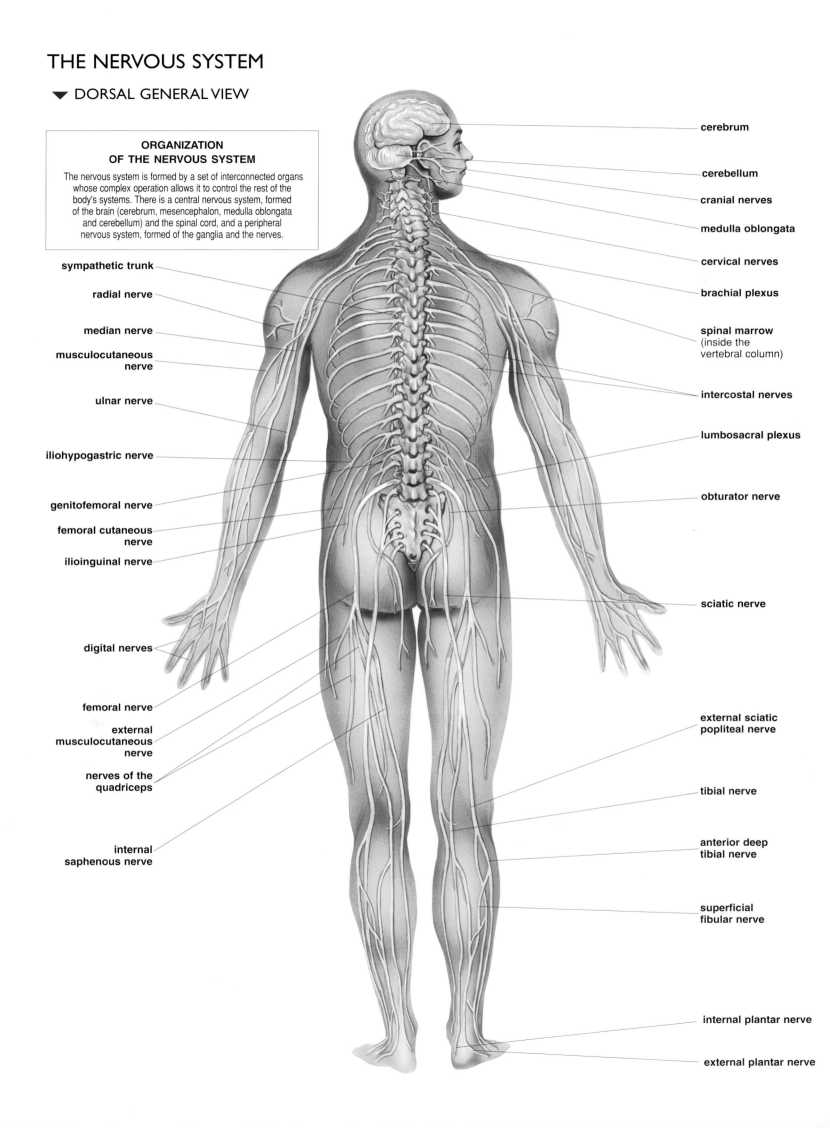

cerebrum

cerebellum

cranial nerves

medulla oblongata

cervical nerves

brachial plexus

spinal marrow
(inside the vertebral column)

intercostal nerves

lumbosacral plexus

obturator nerve

sciatic nerve

external sciatic popliteal nerve

tibial nerve

anterior deep tibial nerve

superficial fibular nerve

internal plantar nerve

external plantar nerve

sympathetic trunk

radial nerve

median nerve

musculocutaneous nerve

ulnar nerve

iliohypogastric nerve

genitofemoral nerve

femoral cutaneous nerve

ilioinguinal nerve

digital nerves

femoral nerve

external musculocutaneous nerve

nerves of the quadriceps

internal saphenous nerve

128

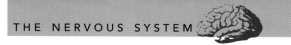

THE AUTONOMIC NERVOUS SYSTEM

AUTONOMIC NERVOUS SYSTEM

The part of the nervous system that regulates the internal activity of the body, controlling the operation of organs such as the heart, blood vessels, the intestines, the kidneys, the different glands, etc. All of these organs act totally independently of the conscious will of the individual. It consists of two parts: the sympathetic system, whose function is to prepare the organism for stressful situations that require alertness; and the parasympathetic system.

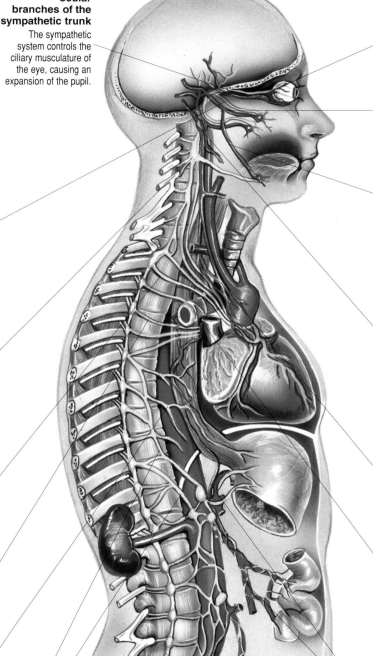

ocular branches of the sympathetic trunk
The sympathetic system controls the ciliary musculature of the eye, causing an expansion of the pupil.

salivary branches of the sympathetic trunk
The sympathetic system acts on the salivary glands by diminishing the salivary secretion. Thus, in situations of fear, in which the sympathetic system is activated, the mouth becomes dry.

sympathetic trunk
A neural chain formed by a succession of ganglia, located on either side of the vertebral column, which extends from the cervical to the lumbar regions. The ganglia receive nerve fibres from the spinal cord, which are connected with the superior centres of control located in the hypothalamus. The ganglia give off nerves which reach the different viscera.

cardiac branches of the sympathetic trunk
The sympathetic system acts on the heart, increasing the frequency and force of the heartbeat and expanding the coronary arteries.

pulmonary branches of the sympathetic trunk
The sympathetic system causes an expansion of the trachea and the bronchi, allowing more air to reach the lungs.

aortic branches of the sympathetic trunk
The sympathetic system controls the operation of the blood vessels, acting to contract them and thus increase blood pressure.

splanchnic branches of the sympathetic trunk
The sympathetic system reaches the stomach and other intestinal organs through the splanchnic branches, causing a reduction of the peristaltic movements, slowing intestinal transit and increasing the muscular tone of the sphincters. The branches act on the kidney by causing a reduction of urine production.

vesical and prostate branches of the sympathetic trunk
The sympathetic system acts on the bladder contracting its sphincter.

oculomotor nerve
The third of the cranial nerves, which contain parasympathetic fibres that control the ciliary musculature of the pupil. The parasympathetic system produces contraction of the pupils.

facial nerve
The seventh cranial pair, which contains some parasympathetic fibres which stimulate the lacrimal, salivary and nasal secretions.

glossopharyngeal nerve
The ninth cranial nerve, which carries some parasympathetic fibres that go to the parotid glands, controlling their secretion.

vagus nerve
Tenth of the cranial nerves, which originates in the medulla oblongata and descends through the neck, thorax and abdomen, sending nervous branches to the different organs of these zones. Most of the fibres of the parasympathetic system pass through the vagus, although some also pass through other cranial pairs.

cardiac branches of the vagus nerve
The parasympathetic system acts on the heart, diminishing the frequency and forces of the heartbeat and contracting the coronary arteries.

pulmonary branches of the vagus nerve
The action of the parasympathetic system on the lung is to contract the tracheal and bronchial musculature.

intestinal branches of the vagus nerve
The parasympathetic system acts on the stomach and intestine through the intestinal branches, increasing peristaltic contractions and accelerating intestinal transit, while simultaneously relaxing the sphincters.

vesical and prostate branches of the vagus nerve
The parasympathetic system relaxes the sphincter of the bladder and stimulates the sexual organs.

129

SYMPATHETIC SYSTEM
(represented in yellow)

PARASYMPATHETIC SYSTEM
(represented in green)

NEURONS

NEURON

The fundamental cell of the nervous tissue, which receives and manufactures information and generates and transmits an answer. It is formed of a cellular body, and prolongations that connect with other neurons and conduct the nervous impulses. According to the shape of the cellular body, neurons can be spherical, polyhedral, star-shaped, conical, etc. Depending on the prolongations they may be unipolar, bipolar or multipolar. The neurons do not regenerate or reproduce, meaning the body's total amount of neurons is fixed from a very young age.

130

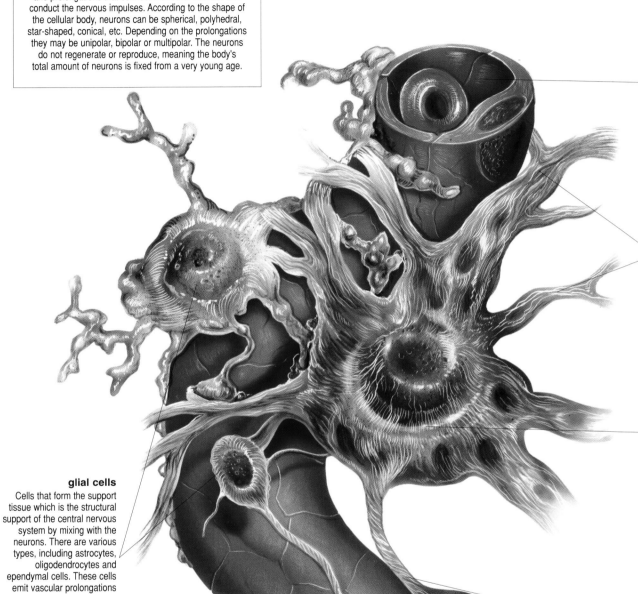

blood capillary
The nervous cells, due to their specific function, have high levels of metabolism. For this reason, their tissue is very rich in blood capillaries, to which the glial cells are attached.

dendrites
Irregularly shaped prolongations of the cytoplasm of the cellular body. They conduct the nervous impulses generated by other neurons to the cellular body. A neuron can have many dendritic prolongations.

cellular body
The central part of the neuron which contains the nucleus. It is surrounded by cytoplasm and the remaining intracellular corpuscles (Golgi apparatus, mitochondria, etc.).

axon
A prolongation of the cellular body with a differentiated structure. The axons constitute most of the nerve fibres and the nerves of the organism. Its function is to conduct the nervous impulse generated in the cellular body to other neurons. Generally, each neuron has a single axon and its length is usually much greater than that of the dendrites.

glial cells
Cells that form the support tissue which is the structural support of the central nervous system by mixing with the neurons. There are various types, including astrocytes, oligodendrocytes and ependymal cells. These cells emit vascular prolongations that adhere to the blood capillaries and the neurons.

Ranvier's nodes
Areas of the axon that are not covered by the myelin sheath.

myelin sheath
Axons are covered by a sheath made of a substance called myelin, which is formed of lipoproteins and produced by some glial cells. It supports the axon and increases the speed of transmission of the nervous impulse.

Schwann cells
Schwann cells are similar in function to oligodendrocytes. They provide myelination to axons in the peripheral nervous system and also have phagocytotic functions.

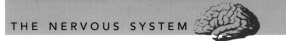

THE STRUCTURE OF A NERVE. SYNAPSE

nerve fibres or axons
Prolongations of the neuron that transport the nervous impulses generated in the central nervous system through the nerves to all parts of the body. Some axons are covered by a myelin sheath and others are not.

nervous fascicle
Groupings of nerve fibres or axons that run through the nerve.

epineurium
A layer of dense connective tissue that covers the nerve.

ganglion
A structure formed by groupings of neuronal bodies located near the spinal marrow and covered by a layer of connective tissue. The ganglia are intermediate stations in the transmission of the nervous impulse from the central nervous system to the periphery.

perineurium
A layer of dense connective tissue located in the interior of the nerve, covering the nervous fascicles.

blood capillaries
The nervous cells, due to their specific function, have high levels of metabolism. For this reason, their tissue is very rich in blood capillaries, to which the glial cells are attached.

endoneurium
A structure formed of loose connective tissue that surrounds and supports the nerve fibres.

nerve
A structure that carries the axons or nerve fibres of the neuronal bodies of the central nervous system or ganglia through the body. Some nerves transmit motor orders (motor nerves), others collect sensory information (sensory nerves) and others carry out both functions (mixed nerves).

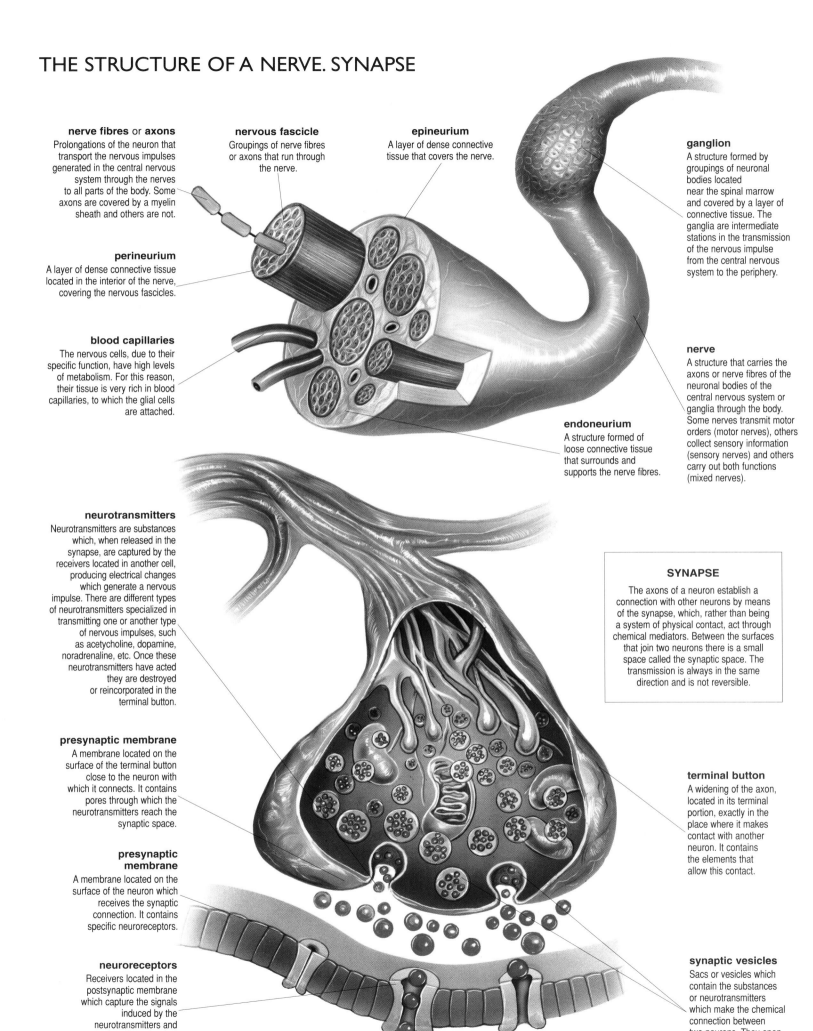

131

neurotransmitters
Neurotransmitters are substances which, when released in the synapse, are captured by the receivers located in another cell, producing electrical changes which generate a nervous impulse. There are different types of neurotransmitters specialized in transmitting one or another type of nervous impulses, such as acetycholine, dopamine, noradrenaline, etc. Once these neurotransmitters have acted they are destroyed or reincorporated in the terminal button.

SYNAPSE

The axons of a neuron establish a connection with other neurons by means of the synapse, which, rather than being a system of physical contact, act through chemical mediators. Between the surfaces that join two neurons there is a small space called the synaptic space. The transmission is always in the same direction and is not reversible.

presynaptic membrane
A membrane located on the surface of the terminal button close to the neuron with which it connects. It contains pores through which the neurotransmitters reach the synaptic space.

terminal button
A widening of the axon, located in its terminal portion, exactly in the place where it makes contact with another neuron. It contains the elements that allow this contact.

presynaptic membrane
A membrane located on the surface of the neuron which receives the synaptic connection. It contains specific neuroreceptors.

neuroreceptors
Receivers located in the postsynaptic membrane which capture the signals induced by the neurotransmitters and turn them into electrical signals that generate nervous impulses.

synaptic vesicles
Sacs or vesicles which contain the substances or neurotransmitters which make the chemical connection between two neurons. They open following the orders of the electrical impulses transmitted by the axons.

THE CEREBRUM

▼ INFERIOR VIEW

frontal lobe
The frontal lobe forms almost all the anterior part of the cerebrum. Its cortical zone performs the majority of intellectual activities of the human being.

sylvian fissure
A fissure that extends from the base of the cerebrum to its external face and separates the frontal and temporal lobes.

optical chiasm
The optical chiasm is formed by the union of the optic nerves and is the site at which fibres from the nasal portion of each retina cross and continue in the opposite optical tract.

stem of the hypophysis
The hypophysis, the gland that is located in the base of the cerebrum, is united with the hypothalamus through this pedicle.

mamillary bodies
Two hemispherical tubercules formed of grey matter. They contain nervous nuclei corresponding to the hypothalamus.

longitudinal cerebral fissure
(anterior part)
A longitudinal fissure in the midline between the two cerebral hemispheres, which extends from the frontal to the occipital pole. The anterior part houses a fibrous wall known as the falx cerebri, so called because of its sickle shape.

olfactory sulci
Two sulci that run across the inferior faces of the frontal lobes. They contain the olfactory tracts.

olfactory tracts
Two nervous cords that communicate the olfactory sensations captured in the nasal fossas to cerebral centres which interpret them. At one end is the olfactory bulb, located above the cribiform lamina of the ethmoid bone, near to the olfactory mucosa of the nasal cavity.

temporal lobe
The temporal lobe is located in the lateral inferior region of each hemisphere. Its cortical zone contains the auditory receptor centres.

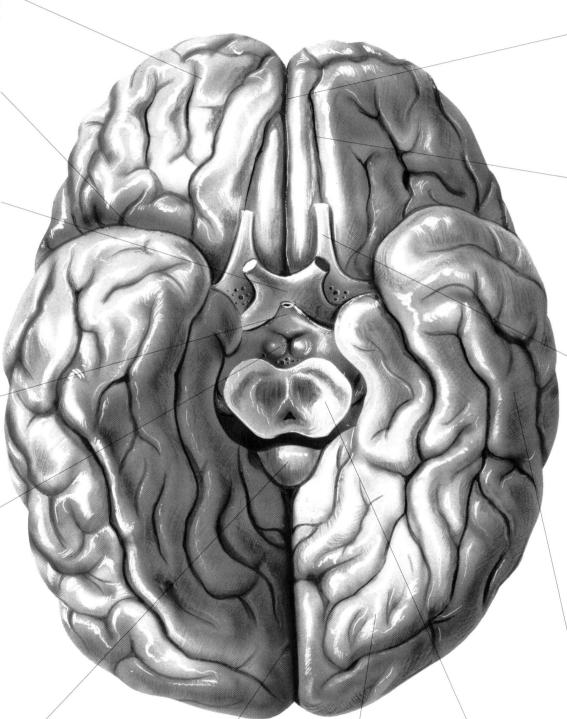

splenium of the corpus callosum
The splenium is the rounded, posterior part of the corpus callosum. It is a lamina of white matter that separates the two cerebral hemispheres.

longitudinal cerebral fissure
(posterior part)
A longitudinal fissure in the midline between the two cerebral hemispheres, which extends from the frontal to the occipital pole.

occipital lobe
The occipital lobe occupies the posterior part of the cerebral hemispheres. Its cortex contains the receptor centres of sight.

cerebral peduncles
Two fibrous columns, united internally, which join the cerebrum and the mesencephalon.

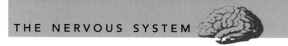

THE CEREBRUM

▼ SUPERIOR VIEW

CEREBRUM

The largest, central part of the nervous system. It receives all conscious and unconscious impressions, and sends out all motor transmissions. In addition, all the intellectual faculties of the human being are concentrated in the superficial cerebral cortex. It is located inside the cranial cavity surrounded by the cranial bones.

left cerebral hemisphere
Left portion of the two into which the cerebrum is divided. Since the nervous routes that descend from the cerebrum to the rest of the body intercross in the zone of the mesencephalon and medulla oblongata, the structures of the left cerebral hemisphere usually dominate over the right in right-handed individuals.

frontal pole
The anterior extreme of the frontal lobe.

right cerebral hemisphere
The cerebrum is divided into right and left lateral hemispheres. The division is external, since in their middle and central portions, the hemispheres are united by the different structures of the base of the cerebrum.

superior frontal sulcus
A sulcus that crosses the antero-external face of the frontal lobe obliquely.

inferior frontal sulcus
A sulcus that runs parallel and inferior to the superior frontal sulcus.

cerebral gyri
The external surface of the two hemispheres is crossed by wide sulci or fissures that delimit the cerebral gyri. This disposition is caused by the necessity to lodge a great amount of cerebral tissue in a closed cavity like the skull. They receive the name of the zone in which they are located: superior central circumvolution, median temporal, precentral, etc.

precentral sulcus
A well-marked sulcus between the cerebral gyri, in front of the central sulcus in the frontal lobe.

central sulcus (Rolando)
A wide fissure that goes from the middle of the interhemispheric fissure perpendicularly, crosses the external face of the cerebral hemispheres, and reaches nearly to the sylvian fissure. It separates the frontal and parietal lobes.

superior temporal sulcus
A sulcus that crosses the superior part of the temporal lobe parallel to the sylvian fissure.

intraparietal sulcus
A sulcus that crosses the parietal lobe and delimits its circumvolutions.

133

postcentral sulcus
A sulcus that separates some of the cerebral gyri of the parietal lobe, following a path parallel to the central sulcus.

longitudinal cerebral fissure
A wide fissure that separates the right and left cerebral hemispheres and extends from the frontal to the occipital poles. In its anterior part it lodges a fibrous wall, the falx cerebri, which is a prolongation of the meningeal layers that cover the cerebrum.

parieto-occipital sulcus
A sulcus that separates the lobes parietal and occipital lobes. It is also called the external perpendicular fissure.

occipital pole
The posterior extreme of the occipital cavity.

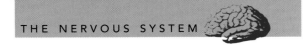

THE CEREBRUM

▼ EXTERNAL LATERAL VIEW

precentral sulcus
A well-marked sulcus between the cerebral gyri, in front of the central sulcus, in the frontal lobe.

central sulcus (Rolando)
A wide fissure that goes from the middle of the interhemispheric fissure perpendicularly, crosses the external surface of the cerebral hemispheres and reaches nearly to the Sylvian fissure. It separates the frontal and parietal lobes.

postcentral sulcus
A sulcus that separates some of the cerebral gyri of the parietal lobe, following a path parallel to the central sulcus.

parieto-occipital sulcus
A sulcus that originates in the posterior third of the interhemispheric sulcus and extends perpendicularly across the superior and external surfaces of the hemispheres. It separates the parietal and occipital lobes.

transverse occipital sulcus
A sulcus that crosses the external surface of the cerebrum vertically, separating the occipital and temporal lobes.

sylvian fissure
A fissure that extends from the base of the cerebrum to its external surface and separates the frontal and temporal lobes.

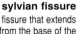

frontal lobe
The frontal lobe forms almost all the anterior part of the cerebrum. It is delimited posteriorly by the central sulcus and inferiorly by the Sylvian fissure. Its cortical zone performs the majority of intellectual activities of the human being, with the motor activities being centred in the gyri anterior to the central sulcus.

parietal lobe
Located in the superior external and central part of the cerebral hemispheres, the parietal lobe is separated from the frontal lobe by the central sulcus and the occipital lobe by the external perpendicular fissure. The sensory receptors from all the body are located in the area posterior to the central sulcus.

temporal lobe
The temporal lobes are located in the infero-lateral region of each hemisphere and are separated from the frontal lobe by the Sylvian fissure and from the occipital lobe by the preoccipital sulcus. They are prolonged in their posterior superior area as the parietal lobes. Their cortical zones contain the auditory receptor centres.

occipital lobe
The occipital lobe occupies the posterior part of the cerebral hemispheres, separated from the temporal lobe by the preoccipital sulcus and the parietal lobe by the external perpendicular sulcus. Its cortex contains the visual receptor centres.

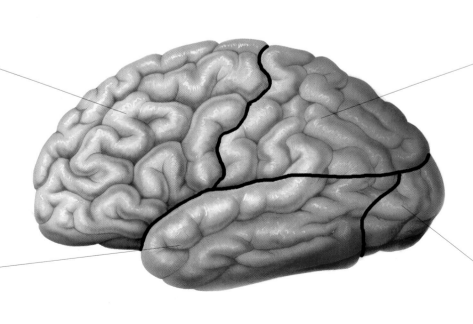

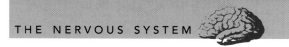

THE CEREBRUM

▼ INTERNAL LATERAL VIEW

septum pelucidum
A medial partition that
extends from the corpus
callosum to the cerebral
trigone and separates the
lateral ventricles.

corpus callosum
The corpus callosum
is a broad, thick
band connecting
both hemispheres and
consisting of a mass of
nerve fibres. It consists
of anterior, medial and
posterior portions.

cerebral trigone
A triangular lamina that
originates in the posterior
part of the corpus callosum
and forms the floor of the
septum pelucidum and the
roof of the third ventricle.

parietal lobe
Located in the superior
external and central
part of the cerebral
hemispheres. The sensory
receptors from all the
body are located in
the area posterior to
the central sulcus.

third ventricle
The third ventricle is a cavity
located below the trigone, whose
lateral walls are formed by the
optical thalamus. It contains the
cerebrospinal fluid which
circulates around the different
ventricles and reaches the
meningeal spaces, where it
protects the cerebrum.

frontal lobe
The frontal lobe forms
almost all the anterior
part of the cerebrum.
It is delimited posteriorly
by the central sulcus
and inferiorly by the
Sylvian fissure. Its
cortical zone performs
the majority of
intellectual activities
of the human being,
with the motor activities
being centred in the
gyri anterior to the
central sulcus.

occipital lobe
The occipital lobe
occupies the posterior
part of the cerebral
hemispheres. Its cortex
contains the visual
receptor centres.

135

optical chiasm
The optic chiasm is
formed by the union
of the optic nerves,
and is the site at
which fibres from
the left optical nerve
cross fibres obliquely
and go to the occipital
lobe of the right
cerebral hemisphere,
and vice versa.

aqueduct of Silvius
A duct that crosses the
cerebral peduncles and
connects the third ventricle
with the fourth ventricle,
located inside the
mesencephalon and
medulla oblongata.

hypophysis
A gland joined to
the cerebrum by the
hypophysial stem which
secretes a series of
hormones that regulate
the operation of the
rest of glands of
the organism.

**cerebral
peduncles**
Two fibrous columns,
joined internally, that
connect join the cerebrum
and the mesencephalon.
They are crossed internally
by the aqueduct of Silvius.

infundibulum
A funnel-shaped
depression located
in the floor of the
third ventricle,
above the
hypophysial stem.

commisura grisea
The commisura grisea
joins the nuclei of the
optical thalami on both
sides of the third ventricle.
It is also called the
interthalamic adherence.

temporal lobe
The temporal lobes are
located in the intero-
lateral area of each of the
hemispheres. The
auditory receptor centres
are located in their
cortical zones.

mamillary bodies
Two hemispherical tubercules,
formed of grey matter.
They contain nuclei which
overlap the hypothalamus.

THE CEREBRUM

▼ LONGITUDINAL SECTION

grey matter
The external layer of the cerebral hemispheres, also called the grey cortex. It contains the neuronal bodies, where the nervous signals are drawn up and information integrated.

lateral ventricles
Two cavities located at each side of the midline of the cerebrum, which extend from the frontal to the occipital lobe. They contain the choroid plexuses which produce the cerebrospinal fluid.

corpus callosum
The corpus callosum is a broad, thick band of white matter connecting both cerebral hemispheres. Its function is to unite the different parts of the hemispheres.

longitudinal cerebral fissure
A longitudinal fissure in the midline between the two cerebral hemispheres, which extends from the frontal to the occipital pole.

septum pelucidum
A medial partition that extends perpendicularly from the inferior part of the corpus callosum to the cerebral trigone and separates the lateral ventricles.

third ventricle
The third ventricle is a cavity located below the lateral ventricles with which it is communicated by the foramen of Monro. It contains the cerebrospinal fluid that circulates around the different ventricles and reaches the meningeal spaces.

caudate nucleus
One of the basal ganglia of the telencephalon or superior cerebrum. It is a nucleus of grey matter located in the wall of the lateral ventricle that constitutes an important link in the transmission of motor impulses.

white matter
A mass of cerebral tissue below the grey cortex, which surrounds the cerebral nuclei. It fundamentally contains nervous elements of transmission and conduction.

Sylvian fissure
A fissure that extends from the base of the cerebrum to its external face and separates the frontal and temporal lobes.

biconvex nucleus
One of the basal ganglia of the telencephalon or superior cerebrum. Like all basal ganglia, it is an important link in the transmission of motor impulses.

optical thalamus
Zones of grey matter located on both sides of the third ventricle, which contains groupings of neurones that serve as a type of relay station of the nervous pathways that connect with the cerebral cortex.

hippocampus
The hippocampus is located inside the temporal lobe. It forms part of the limbic system and plays a role in memory and direction.

cerebral peduncles
Two fibrous columns, united internally, that join the cerebrum and the mesencephalon. They contain nerves that enter and leave the cerebrum.

mamillary bodies
Two hemispherical tubercules formed of grey matter. They contain nervous nuclei corresponding to the hypothalamus.

cranial nerves
The seventh (facial), eighth (vestibulocochlear), ninth (glossopharyngeal), tenth (vagus) and twelfth (hypoglossal) nerves which leave the lateral walls of the bulb and the sulcus that separates it from the mesencephalon

mesencephalon
An eminence located between the medulla oblongata and the base of the cerebrum, with which it is connected by the cerebral peduncles. It contains the nervous pathways that communicate the cerebrum with the spinal marrow. Its centre contains a cavity called the fourth ventricle.

medulla oblongata
The superior, thicker portion of the spinal cord. It leaves the cranial cavity through the occipital foramen. It contains the nervous pathways that unite the cerebrum with the spinal cord. It also contains the centres that regulate breathing and the circulation.

cerebellum
The cerebellum is located below the occipital lobes of the cerebrum and behind the protuberance, in the occipital cerebellar fossa. It is formed by one medial and two lateral lobes. Its main function is to coordinate the movements of many skeletal muscles of the body, and is thus essential for the maintenance of posture, balance and gait, etc.

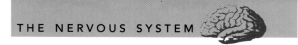

THE CEREBRUM

▼ CROSS-SECTION

septum pelucidum
A medial partition that extends from the corpus callosum to the cerebral trigone and separates the lateral ventricles.

caudate nucleus
One of the basal ganglia of the telencephalon or superior cerebrum. It is a nucleus of grey matter located in the wall of the lateral ventricle that constitutes an important link in the transmission of motor impulses.

longitudinal cerebral fissure
(anterior part)
A longitudinal fissure in the midline between the two cerebral hemispheres, which contains the fibrous wall called the falx cerebri.

genu of the corpus callosum
The anterior part of the corpus callosum which consists of a lamina of white matter between both cerebral hemispheres, which it connects.

biconvex nucleus
One of the basal ganglia of the telencephalon or superior cerebrum. Like all of them, it constitutes an important link in the transmission of motor impulses.

anterior horns of the lateral ventricles
The anterior zones of the lateral ventricles. The anterior horns extend from the frontal lobe to the occipital lobe. The anterior horns or prolongations are located in the sinus of the frontal lobes. They contain the cerebrospinal fluid.

optical thalamus
Zones of grey matter that contain groupings of nervous cells that serve as a type of relay station of the nervous pathways that connect with the cerebral cortex.

grey matter
The external layer of the cerebral hemispheres, also called the grey cortex. Grey matter is also found in the interior of the brain in the different nuclei or specialized nervous groupings. It contains the neuronal bodies, where the nervous signals are drawn up and information integrated.

white matter
A mass of cerebral tissue below the grey cortex which surrounds the cerebral nuclei. It fundamentally contains nervous elements of transmission and conduction.

third ventricle
The third ventricle is a cavity located below the lateral ventricles with which it is communicated by the foramen of Monro. It contains the cerebrospinal fluid which circulates around the different ventricles and reaches the meningeal spaces.

central sulcus (Rolando)
A wide fissure that extends perpendicularly from the middle of the interhemispheric fissure and crosses the external face of the cerebral hemispheres.

occipital horns of the lateral ventricles
Posterior parts of the lateral ventricles located in the occipital lobe. The ventricles contain the cerebrospinal fluid.

longitudinal cerebral fissure
(posterior part)
A wide fissure that separates the right and left cerebral hemispheres and extends from the frontal to the occipital poles.

splenium of the corpus callosum
The splenium is the rounded, posterior part of the corpus callosum which separates the two cerebral hemispheres.

choroid plexus
Cord-like formations that are prolongations of the meninges and are located in the frontal and occipital horns of the lateral ventricles. Their function is to secrete cerebrospinal fluid.

ORIGIN OF THE CRANIAL NERVES

▼ INFERIOR VIEW

oculomotor nerve (III cranial nerve)
The nerve that transmits motor orders to all the ocular musculature. It originates in the cerebral peduncles and enters the ocular cavity through the orbital fissure.

trochlear nerve (IV cranial nerve)
A nerve with a long intracranial passage from its origin in the lateral zone of the cerebral peduncles to its termination in the ocular cavity. It ends in the greater oblique muscle of the eye, whose operations it controls.

trigeminal nerve (V cranial nerve)
A nerve that receives the sensations of the face, orbit, oral cavity and the nasal fossas and transmits the motor orders to the chewing muscles. It originates in the mesencephalon, where a knot, called the ganglion of Gasser, forms and from which emerge its three branches, the ophthalmic, maxillary and mandibular.

facial nerve (VII cranial nerve)
A sensory motor nerve that originates in the pontomedullary sulcus. It has two branches, a motor root and a sensory root called the nervus intermedius. It goes laterally towards the internal acoustic duct, crosses the petrous bone and emits tympanic, auricular, lingual, temporal, facial and cervical branches and others to the parotid gland.

nervus intermedius
A sensory branch of the facial nerve that innervates the lingual, sublingual and submaxillary glands.

vestibulocochlear nerve (VIII cranial nerve)
A sensory nerve that originates in the pontomedullary sulcus and penetrates in the internal acoustic duct. It transmits auditory sensations and other postural transmissions that help to maintain the balance.

glossopharyngeal nerve (IX cranial nerne)
A sensory motor nerve that originates in the medulla oblongata. It exits the skull through the posterior jugular foramen and has branches, some of which unite with the facial nerve and others that go to the tympanic cavity, penetrating in the petrous bone, towards the carotid zone, lingual and pharyngeal and innervating some of the pharyngeal muscles.

optical nerve (II cranial nerve)
The optical nerves are two nervous structures that transport the visual sensations collected in the terminations of the ocular retina to the interior of the brain.

olfactory tracts
Two nervous cords that communicate the olfactory sensations captured in the nasal fossae to cerebral centres that interpret them. At one end is the olfactory bulb, located above the cribiform lamina of the ethmoid bone, near to the olfactory mucosa of the nasal cavity, to which are united the nerve fibres that constitute the two olfactory or first cranial nerves.

abducent nerve (VI cranial nerve)
An exclusively motor nerve, that originates in the sulcus that separates the mesencephalon from the medulla oblongata. It goes to the ocular cavity from where it supplies the rectus lateralis muscle of the eye.

mesencephalon
An eminence located between the medulla oblongata and the base of the cerebrum, with which it is connected by the cerebral peduncles. It contains the nervous pathways that communicate the cerebrum with the spinal cord.

medulla oblongata
The superior, thicker portion of the spinal cord which contains the internal nuclei that originate various cranial nerves. It also contains the centres that regulate breathing and the circulation.

hypoglossal nerve (XII cranial nerve)
Motor nerve that originates in the lateral zone of the bulb and innervates a large part of the lingual musculature.

cerebellum
An intracranial organ located below the occipital lobes of the brain, behind the mesencephalon and over the medulla oblongata. Its main function is to coordinate the movements of many of the skeletal muscles of the body.

vagus nerve (X cranial nerve)
A sensory motor nerve that originates in the medulla oblongata; it leaves the cranial cavity by the jugular foramen and descends through the neck and thorax to the abdomen, emitting many nervous branches in its path.

spinal medulla
A long, almost cylindrical cord that is the continuation of the medulla oblongata and descends down the back, contained by the spinal column or vertebral column. It contains the spinal nerves that go to all parts of the body.

spinal or accessory nerve (XI cranial nerve)
A sensory motor nerve formed by the union of several nervous branches that originate in the medulla oblongata and the spinal marrow. It supplies the soft palate, larynx, pharynx and the trapezius and sternocleidomastoid muscles, and has a branch that unites with the vagus nerve.

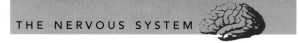

THE CEREBELLUM

▼ POSTERIOR VIEW

superior vermis
A swelling that constitutes the central lobe of the cerebellum, located between the two cerebellar hemispheres.

cerebellar hemispheres
The two lateral lobes of the cerebellum. Their surface is marked by a series of parallel sulci.

CEREBELLUM
An intracranial organ located below the occipital lobes of the brain and behind the pons and medulla oblongata lodged in the posterior cranial fossa. It is composed of two lateral lobes and a medial lobe. Its main function is to coordinate the movements of the skeletal muscles of the body, and it is vital for functions such as maintenance of the bodily position, the balance, etc.

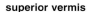

▼ ANTERIOR VIEW

fourth ventricle
The posterior wall of the fourth ventricle is formed by a lamina called the tectorial membrane, which is attached to the anterior face of the cerebellum.

cerebellar peduncles
Structures that unite the cerebellum with the mesencephalon. Bunches of nerve fibres that connect both parts of the nervous system run through them. There are superior, medial and inferior peduncles.

fissures of the cerebellum
Multiple fissures that furrow all the surface of the cerebellum. They penetrate more or less deeply in the cerebellar tissue.

inferior vermis
The vermis extends across the inferior face of the cerebellum, maintaining a constant shape.

139

horizontal fissure
A sulcus that divides the anterior face of the cerebellar hemispheres in superior and inferior parts.

▼ HORIZONTAL CROSS-SECTION

fourth ventricle
A cavity located between the mesencephalon and the cerebellum, it runs between the two cerebellar peduncles. It is also called the rhomboid fossa, and it contains the cerebrospinal fluid.

vermis
The central lobe of the cerebellum which runs from front to back. It is composed of various zones known as the lingual, pyramid, uvula, nodule and tuber vermis.

cerebellar cortex
A thin layer of grey matter, that is very rich in neurons, and comprises the external part of the cerebellum, covering all the cerebellar sulci and elevations.

cerebellar nuclei
Structures composed of grey matter located in the sinus of the cerebellar tissue. They are classified as dentate, globose, emboliform and fastigial nuclei. They receive nerve fibres from the cerebellar cortex and emit others that go to other parts of the nervous system.

medullar substance
A white substance, formed by nervous prolongations of the neurons located in the grey matter of the cortex.

THE MEDULLA OBLONGATA AND MESENCEPHALON

▼ ANTERIOR VIEW

cerebral peduncles
Two fibrous columns, united internally, that join the cerebrum and the mesencephalon.

oculomotor nerve (III cranial nerve)
The nerve that transmits motor orders to all the ocular musculature.

olfactory tract
A nervous termination that communicates the olfactory sensations captured in the nasal fossas to the cerebral centres that interpret them.

optical chiasm
The optical chiasm is formed by the union of the optic nerves and is the site at which fibres from the left optical nerve cross fibres obliquely and go to the occipital lobe of the right cerebral hemisphere, and vice versa.

stem of the hypophysis
The hypophysis, the gland that is located in the base of the cerebrum in the cavity of the sphenoid bone called the sella turcica, is united with the hypothalamus through this pedicle.

mamillary bodies
Two hemispherical tubercules, formed of grey matter. They contain nervous nuclei corresponding to the hypothalamus.

trochlear nerve (IV cranial nerve)
A motor nerve that goes to the orbit and is responsible for the mobility of the greater oblique muscle of the eye.

trigeminal nerve (V cranial nerve)
A mixed nerve (motor and sensory) that receives transmissions from the face, orbit, oral cavity and nasal fossas, and transmits motor orders to the chewing muscles. It has three branches: the ophthalmic, maxilla and mandibular nerves.

mesencephalon
The mesencephalon is located between the medulla oblongata and the base of the brain. It connects with the brain through the cerebral peduncles. It contains the nerves that communicate the brain with the spinal marrow.

abducent nerve (VI cranial nerve)
A motor nerve that goes to the ocular cavity and innervates the external rectum muscle of the eye.

pontomedullary sulcus
A sulcus that separates the mesencephalon from the medulla oblongata.

medulla oblongata
The superior, thicker portion of the spinal marrow. Its interior contains the nerves that unite the brain with the spinal marrow. It also contains the centres that regulate breathing and the circulation.

anterior medial sulcus
A sulcus that crosses the anterior surface of the medulla oblongata and extends down the spinal marrow in the same direction.

hypoglossal nerve (XII cranial nerve)
A motor muscle that innervates a large part of the lingual musculature.

spinal or accessory nerve (XI cranial nerve)
A sensory motor nerve that emits ramifications to the villi of the palate, larynx, pharynx and to the trapezius and sternocleidomastoid muscles.

cerebellum
An intracranial organ located below the occipital lobes of the brain, behind the mesencephalon and over the medulla oblongata. Its main function is to coordinate the movements of many multiple skeletal muscles of the body, making it essential for the body's posture and balance.

vagus nerve (X cranial nerve)
A sensory motor nerve that leaves the cranial cavity and descends through the neck and thorax to the abdomen, emitting many nervous branches in its path.

facial nerve (VII cranial nerve)
A sensory motor nerve that has two branches: the proper facial nerve and the sensory nerve that is the intermediate nerve that innervates the lingual, sublingual and submaxillary glands.

vestibulocochlear nerve (VIII cranial nerve)
A sensory nerve that transmits auditory sensations to the cochlear area and collects sensations from the vestibular area of the ear which help to maintain the balance.

glossopharyngeal nerve (IX cranial nerve)
A sensory motor nerve that emits nervous terminations, some of which go to be united with the facial nerve and others that go to the tympanic cavity and the carotid, lingual and pharyngeal areas.

THE MEDULLA OBLONGATA AND MESENCEPHALON

▼ INTERNAL VIEW

commisura grisea
The commisura grisea joins the nuclei of the optical thalami on both sides of the third ventricle. It is also called the interthalamic adherence.

third ventricle
The third ventricle is a cavity located below the lateral ventricles with which it is connected by the foramen of Monro. It contains the cerebrospinal fluid that circulates around the different ventricles and reaches the meningeal spaces.

corpus callosum
The corpus callosum is a broad, thick band of white matter located between the cerebral hemispheres which connects the different areas of the hemispheres.

aqueduct of Silvius
A duct that crosses the cerebral peduncles and communicates the third ventricle with the fourth ventricle, allowing the cerebrospinal fluid to flow between the two spaces.

mamillary tubercules
Two half-moon-shaped papilla formed of grey matter. They contain nervous nuclei corresponding to the hypothalamus.

pineal gland or epiphysis
A gland located in the posterior wall of the third ventricle that secretes a hormone known as melatonin.

optical chiasm
The optical chiasm is formed by the union of the optic nerves and is the site at which fibres from the left optical nerve cross obliquely and go to the occipital lobe of the right cerebral hemisphere, and vice versa.

quadrigeminal bodies
Four tubercules, located in the posterior face of the mesencephalon, that contain nervous nuclei that take part in the transmission of the visual and auditory sensations.

hypophysis
A gland joined to the cerebrum by the hypophysial stem which secretes a series of hormones that regulate the operation of the rest of the glands of the organism.

cerebellum
An intracranial organ located behind the mesencephalon and above the medulla oblongata. It is composed of two lateral lobes and a medial lobe. Its main function is to coordinate the movements of the skeletal muscles and it is vital for the maintenance of the posture and balance.

mesencephalon
An eminence located between the medulla oblongata and the cerebral peduncles. It contains the nervous pathways that coonnect the cerebrum with the spinal marrow.

medulla oblongata
The superior, thicker portion of the spinal marrow. Its interior contains the nerves that unite the brain with the spinal marrow. It also contains the centres that regulate breathing and the circulation.

fourth ventricle
A cavity located between the mesencephalon and the cerebellum, in which the aqueduct of Silvius, coming from the medial ventricle, ends. It continues inferiorly as the central medullary duct. The cerebrospinal fluid circulates in the fourth ventricle and goes to the subarchnoid space of the meninges through orifices located in the lateral face of the fourth ventricle.

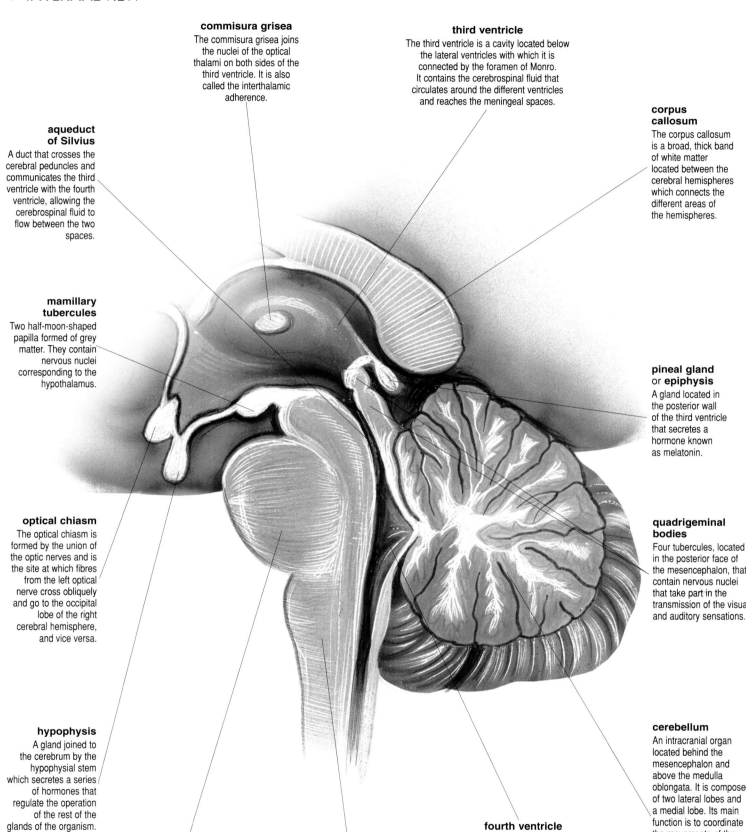

141

SPINAL CORD

SPINAL MEDULLA

Part of the central nervous system which leaves the cranial cavity and crosses the trunk vertically through the vertebral column. It is almost cylindrical and sends out nerves that go to all parts of the body.

medulla oblongata

The superior, thicker portion of the spinal marrow. It contains the nervous pathways that unite the brain with the spinal marrow. It also contains the vital centers which regulate breathing and the circulation.

phrenic nerve

A nerve that originates in the cervical plexus and descends down the neck and thorax to reach the diaphragm which it innervates.

spinal nerves

Lateral branches are emitted by the spinal cord throughout all its length. They leave the vertebral column through the intervertebral foramens. The spinal nerves innervate all the areas of the body. These nerves are divided into anterior and posterior branches immediately after leaving the vertebral column. There are 31 pairs of spinal nerves: eight cervical, twelve thoracic, five lumbar, five sacral and one coccygeal.

intercostal nerve

All the spinal nerves divide into anterior and posterior branches. The anterior branches of the thoracic spinal nerves follow a path parallel to the ribs, in the intercostal spaces and are thus called the intercostal nerves. They innervate the intercostal muscles, and the last intercostal nerves also innervate the muscles of the abdominal wall.

conus medullaris

The conical shape adopted by the medullar cylinder in its final part, after tending to sharpen. It continues as the terminal filum.

cauda equina

A bunch of nervous cords that descend vertically and obliquely from the medullar cone. It is formed by the nervous roots of the three last lumbar spinal nerves and the sacral and coccygeal nerves.

spinal dura mater

The spinal marrow is covered, as are other parts of the central nervous system, by the meninges, which are three membranous layers, called, externally to internally, the dura mater, arachnoid membrane and pia mater. The dura mater extends downwards, beyond the spinal cord, and forms a pouch that reaches the second sacral vertebra.

cerebellum

An intracranial organ located behind the mesencephalon and above the medulla oblongata. It is composed of two lateral lobes and a medial lobe. Its main function is to coordinate the movements of the skeletal muscles, and it is vital for the maintenance of balance.

posterior medial sulcus

A sulcus that crosses the posterior face of the spinal cord vertically, beginning in the medulla oblongata and terminating in the sacral area.

cervical plexus

The cervical plexus is formed by the union of the anterior branches of the first four cervical spinal nerves, which give rise to a series of nervous ramifications that innervate all the structures of the neck.

brachial plexus

The brachial plexus is formed by the union of the anterior branches of the fifth, sixth, seventh and eighth cervical spinal nerves, and the first thoracic nerve, which give rise to three thick nervous trunks, from which come the nerves that innervate the superior extremity.

vertebral pedicles

The bony walls of the vertebral foramen through which the spinal nerves pass.

intervertebral foramini

Orifices delimited by the vertebral pedicles, through which the different somatic nerves emerge from the vertebral column.

subcostal nerve

The last of the intercostal nerves. It does not pass between two ribs but under the last rib. It follows a path similar to the intercostal nerves and descends to the gluteal region.

lumbosacral plexus

A plexus formed by the union of the anterior branches of the lumbar spinal nerves and those of the first three sacral nerves. It innervates all the inferior extremity, the inferior abdominal area and the genital area.

terminal filum

A thin, rudimentary prolongation of the conus medullaris which is inserted in the coccyx.

142

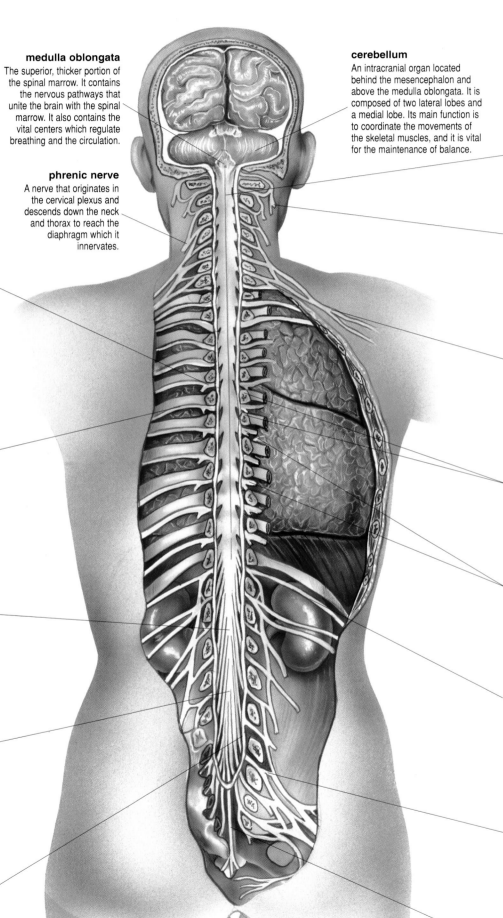

THE MENINGES

superior longitudinal sinus
A venous duct in the dura mater crosses the cerebral interhemispheric area from front to back.

scalp
The layer of skin that covers the skull and is generally covered by hair.

subcutaneous cellular tissue
Deep in the skin it contains much fatty tissue that serves to cushion and protect the deeper structures.

skull
The bony structure that surrounds the brain. It is formed of two laminae called diploe that surround a central area of spongy tissue.

dura mater
The external, thickest layer of the meninges. It is attached to the periosteum or internal layer of the cranial bone. It has a fibrous structure and its function is to protect the cerebral structures and maintain them in position.

MENINGES
Layers that cover the central nervous system from the brain to the spinal marrow. There are three layers: the dura mater, the arachnoid membrane and the pia mater.

meningeal arteries and veins
A dense network of arteries and veins that run through the meninges. The arteries come from three main branches: the anterior, median and posterior meningeal arteries. The veins go to the venous sinuses that surround the brain.

subdural space
The space between the dura mater and the arachnoid membrane. It is a very narrow space, almost non-existent in parts, as the two meningeal layers are attached to each other over a large part of their surface. The meningeal veins, arteries and nerves pass through the space.

arachnoid membrane
A thin, fibrous membrane that is attached to the internal face of the dura mater and has a similar extension.

subarachnoid space
A somewhat wider space between the arachnoid membrane and the pia mater. The two membranes are not attached to each other, making the subarachnoid space wider. It contains cerebrospinal fluid, whose main function is to protect the brain from any impact.

143

falx cerebri
A fibrous prolongation of the dura mater, which is contained in the longitudinal fissure and separates the cerebral hemispheres.

white matter
A mass of cerebral tissue located below the cerebral cortex which surrounds the different cerebral nuclei. It mainly contains nervous elements of transmission and conduction.

cerebral cortex
The superficial part of the brain, located immediately below the piameter, is an area formed of grey matter, which contains many neurons with specific functions. The cerebral cortex contains the mechanisms responsible for memory, the elaboration of thought, manual skills, speech, etc.

pia mater
The internal layer of the meninges, which is attached to the external surface of the brain, cerebellum, spinal marrow, etc. and covers all the irregularities produced on the surface of these organs.

THE LUMBOSACRAL PLEXUS

LUMBOSACRAL PLEXUS

A plexus formed by the union of the anterior branches of the lumbar spinal nerves and those of the three first sacral nerves. It innervates all the inferior extremity, the inferior abdominal area and the genital area.

ilioinguinal nerve

It originates from the anterior branch of the first lumbar spinal nerve. It follows a similar path to the iliohypogastric nerve and collaborates with it in the innervation of the inferior abdomen and the genital area.

lateral cutaneous nerve thigh

A nerve that is formed from the anterior branches of the second and third lumbar spinal nerves. It follows a descending path and leaves the abdominal cavity passing below the inguinal ligament. In the inferior extremity, it divides into an anterior or femoral branch and a posterior or gluteal branch, which innervate the superficial cutaneous zones of these regions.

genitofemoral nerve

A nerve that originates in the anterior branch of the second lumbar spinal nerve. It bifurcates into the external or femoral branch, which crosses the inguinal ligament and goes to the superior part of the thigh, and the internal or genital branch which goes through the inguinal canal to the scrotum in men and the labia majora in women.

femoral nerve

A thick nerve that originates in the union of the anterior branches of the second, third and fourth lumbar spinal nerves. It goes to the inferior extremity through the inguinal ligament and divides into four branches: the external and internal musculocutaneous nerves, the quadriceps nerve and the internal saphenous nerve.

subcostal nerve

The last of the intercostal nerves. It does not pass between two ribs but under the last rib. It does not belong to the lumbosacral plexus but follows a path similar to the intercostal nerves, descending to the gluteal region.

iliohypogastric nerve

It originates in the anterior branch of the first lumbar spinal nerve and gives rise to branches that supply the gluteal region, the inferior zone of the abdominal wall, and others descend through the inguinal canal to the genital area and the superior part of the thigh.

sympathetic trunk

A part of the autonomic nervous system. It is formed by a series of joined nervous ganglia that run down the vertebral column from the thoracic cavity to the abdominal cavity, supplying organs of these regions.

lumbosacral trunk

The result of the union of the anterior branches of the fourth and fifth lumbar spinal nerves. It descends to unite with the anterior branches of the first spinal sacral nerves to form the sciatic nerve.

pudendal nerves

Nerves that originate in the union of the anterior branches of the second and third spinal sacral nerves. They descend to the genital zone, where they send branches to the perineum and to the penis in men and the clitoris in women.

anal nerve

A nerve that originates in the union of the anterior branches of the third and fourth spinal sacral nerves and follows a parallel path to the pudendal nerve, finally reaching the anal region.

inguinal ligament

A thin, fibrous ligament that extends obliquely from the anterosuperior iliac spine to the pubis. It marks the limit between the pelvic and femoral regions. The vessels and nerves that go to the inferior extremity pass under the inguinal ligament.

sciatic nerve

The largest nerve in the body. It originates in the union of the lumbosacral trunk with the anterior branches of the first spinal sacral nerves. It leaves the pelvis through the greater sciatic notch and, after passing behind the hip joint, it descends the posterior part of the thigh, dividing into two branches at the height of the popliteal fossa of the knee: the libial and common peroneal nerves.

accessory obturator nerve

A nerve that follows a parallel path to the obturator nerve but is not present in all people.

obturator nerve

A nerve formed by the union of the anterior branches of the second, third and fourth lumbar spinal nerves. It descends to the pelvic cavity where it divides into different branches that supply the adductor muscles of the thigh.

THE BRACHIAL PLEXUS

BRACHIAL PLEXUS

The brachial plexus is formed by the union of the anterior branches of the fifth, sixth, seventh and eighth cervical spinal nerves and the first thoracic nerve. It gives rise to the superior, middle and inferior trunks, which are the origin of all the nerves going to the superior extremity.

musculocutaneous nerve

A nerve that originates in the superior trunk of the brachial plexus. It crosses the external part of the arm and the forearm, giving motor branches to the muscles of the anterior face of the arm and sensory branches to the skin of the forearm, where some of its terminal branches arrive to the wrist (lateral antebrachial cutaneous nerve).

radial nerve

A nerve that originates in the middle trunk of the brachial plexus. It goes to the axilla, passes along the posterior aspect of the arm, crossing it behind the humerus, and at the elbow divides into an anterior or sensory branch and a posterior or muscular branch. In its path down the arm the radial nerve sends muscular branches to the triceps and other muscles of the zone, and sensory branches to the skin (posterior antebrachial cutaneous nerve).

superior trunk

Formed by the union of the anterior branches of the fifth and sixth spinal nerves, with a small branch from the fourth. The superior trunk originates the musculocutaneous nerve and part of the median nerve. A posterior branch joins the middle trunk to give rise to the radial nerve.

axillary (circumflex) nerve

A nerve that originates in the middle trunk of the brachial plexus, from which the radial nerve emerges. It separates from the path of the radial nerve and, after crossing below the shoulder joint, it terminates in that area, sending articular branches for the shoulder joint, motor branches to the deltoid muscle and others, and sensory branches to the skin of the shoulder.

middle trunk

The middle trunk originates exclusively in the anterior root of the seventh cervical spinal nerve. Near the axilla, it emits a branch that is united to the prolongation of the superior trunk. The middle trunk has a posterior branch which originates the radial nerve.

inferior trunk

Its origin is in the union of the anterior branches of the eighth cervical spinal nerve and the first thoracic. It gives rise to the medial cutaneous nerves of the arm and forearm. It also has a branch that contributes to forming the median nerve and another posterior branch that originates the radial nerve.

145

long thoracic nerve

A nerve that originates in the small posterior branches of the fifth, sixth and seventh spinal nerves and descends vertically towards the lateral wall of the thorax to innervate the anterior serratus muscle.

pectoral nerves

Anterior collateral branches of the brachial plexus that innervate the greater and smaller pectoral muscles.

subscapular nerves

Posterior collateral branches of the brachial plexus which innervate the subscapular and teres major muscles.

median nerve

The median nerve originates at the height of the axilla through the union of branches of the superior and inferior trunks. It descends along the medial border of the anterior face of the arm, crosses the elbow joint and continues in the central zone of the anterior face of the forearm, crossing the wrist and terminating in the palm of the hand. It emits the majority of its muscular and sensory branches in the forearm and the hand, sending out only some branches to the humerus and the elbow joint in the arm.

ulnar nerve

A nerve that originates in the inferior trunk of the brachial plexus, passes along the medial border of the arm and the elbow and extends down the forearm to the hand. It has no branches in the upper arm. In the forearm it gives rise to branches that go to the elbow joint and the medial muscles of the anterior forearm.

medial antebrachial cutaneous nerve

A nerve that originates in the same trunk as the ulnar nerve and descends parallel to it down the arm. After crossing the elbow, it distributes in multiple sensory branches in the medial surface of the forearm.

medial cutaneous nerve of the arm

A nerve that originates in the same trunk as the ulnar nerve, above the medial antebrachial cutaneous nerve, and descends with these two nerves to terminate in a series of sensory branches that go to the internal and posterior areas of the skin of the arm.

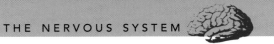

ARM

axillary (circumflex humeral) nerve
A nerve that originates in the middle trunk of the brachial plexus, from which the radial nerve emerges. It separates from the path of the radial nerve and, after crossing below the shoulder joint, it terminates in that area, sending articular branches to the shoulder joint, motor branches to the deltoid muscle, and sensory branches to the skin of the shoulder.

musculocutaneous nerve
A nerve that originates in the brachial plexus formed from the union of the fifth and sixth spinal nerves. It crosses the external part of the arm and forearm, giving motor branches to the anterior muscles of the arm and sensory branches to the skin of the forearm. Some of its terminal branches reach the wrist (lateral antebrachial cutaneous nerve).

posterior cutaneous nerve of the forearm
A branch of the radial nerve that supplies the skin of the posterior forearm.

radial nerve
A nerve that originates in the brachial plexus from the union of the sixth, seventh and eighth cervical nerves and the first thoracic nerve. It runs through the axilla, then down the posterior surface of the arm, crossing it behind the humerus, and at the elbow divides into an anterior or sensory branch and a posterior or muscular branch. In its path down the arm the radial nerve sends muscular branches to the triceps and other muscles of the zone, and sensory branches to the skin (posterior antebrachial cutaneous nerve).

lateral cutaneous nerve of the forearm
A prolongation of the musculocutaneous nerve in the forearm, which it reaches by the anterior face of the elbow joint. Here it sends multiple sensory terminations to the skin of the external face of the forearm and the wrist.

medial cutaneous nerve of the arm
A nerve that originates in the same trunk as the ulnar nerve, above the medial antebrachial cutaneous nerve, and descends with these two nerves to terminate in a series of branches that go to the internal posterior area of the skin of the arm.

medial cutaneous nerve of the forearm
A nerve that originates in the same trunk as the ulnar nerve and descends parallel to it down the arm. After crossing the elbow, it is distributes multiple sensory branches to the medial surface of the forearm.

ulnar nerve
A nerve that originates in the brachial plexus from the union of the eighth cervical and first thoracic nerve. It crosses the medial border of the arm and the elbow and extends down the forearm to the hand. It has no branches in the upper arm.

median nerve
A nerve that originates in the brachial plexus from the union of the sixth, seventh and eighth cervical and first thoracic spinal nerves. It descends the anterior surface of the arm, crosses the elbow joint and continues in the central zone of the anterior surface of the forearm, crossing the wrist and terminating in the palm of the hand. It emits the majority of its muscular and sensory branches in the forearm and the hand, sending out only some branches to the humerus and the elbow joint in the arm.

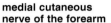
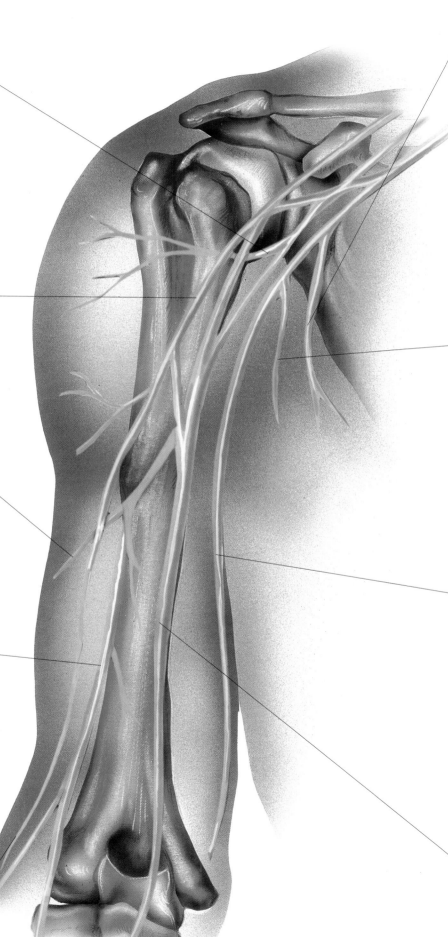

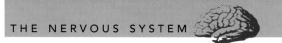

THE FOREARM AND HAND

lateral forearm cutaneous nerve
A prolongation of the musculocutaneous nerve in the forearm, which it reaches through the anterior face of the elbow joint. Once in this zone, it branches into multiple sensory terminations that reach the skin of the external face of the forearm and the wrist.

radial nerve
After crossing the posterior face of the arm, where it has muscular and sensory branches, the radial nerve reaches the elbow, which it crosses laterally, to reach the forearm, where it divides into two branches, one superficial sensory branch and another deep muscular branch.

superficial terminal branch of the radial nerve
The radial nerve divides into two muscular branches when it reaches the forearm. The superficial terminal branch crosses the posteroexternal part of the forearm. It descends to innervate the external dorsal surface of the hand.

deep terminal branch of the radial nerve
The radial nerve divides into two muscular branches when it reaches the forearm. The deep terminal branch sends branches to the posterior muscles of the posterior face of the forearm.

common palmar digital nerves
When it reaches the palm of the hand, the median nerve emits different branches that innervate the muscles of the thenar eminence and the palm of the hand. It has branches to the first, second, third and fourth fingers.

palmar digital nerves
The palmar digital branches of the median nerve innervate the first, second, third and lateral side of the fourth finger

median nerve
The median nerve descends the arm, crosses the elbow joint and continues in the centre of the anterior part of the forearm, crossing the wrist and terminating in the palm of the hand. It emits the majority of its muscular and sensory branches in the area of the forearm, innervating the anterior muscles of the forearm. After crossing the wrist, it divides into several branches that go to the fingers.

anterior interosseal nerve
A branch of this median nerve that passes to the interosseal space located between the ulna and radius and innervates the muscles of the space.

ulnar nerve
The ulnar nerve crosses the medial border of the arm and the elbow behind the epitrochlea and extends down the forearm to the hand. In its path down the arm it has no branches. In the forearm it gives rise to nervous branches that go to the elbow joint and the muscles of the medial forearm and, after crossing the wrist, sends a sensory branch to the dorsal face of the hand and emits deep and superficial terminal branches.

deep terminal branch of the ulnar nerve
The ulnar nerve bifurcates into two branches when it reaches the palm of the hand. The deep branch goes transversally to the thumb, innervating some muscles of the little finger, the thumb and the interosseal spaces.

superficial terminal branch of the ulnar nerve
A more medial branch which goes to the hypothenar eminence where it emits digital branches that go to the fourth and fifth fingers.

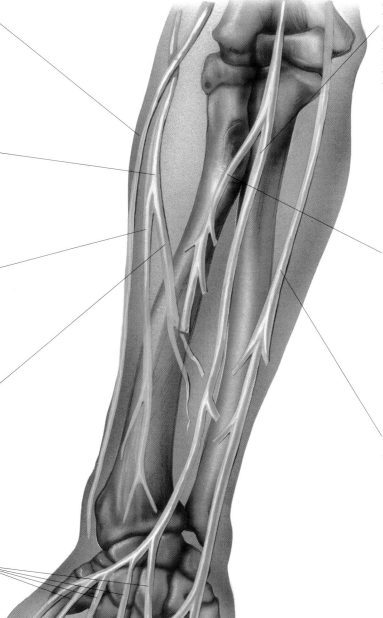

147

THE LEG AND FOOT

sciatic nerve
The largest nerve in the body. It originates in the union of the lumbosacral trunk with the anterior branches of the first spinal sacral nerves. It leaves the pelvis through the greater sciatic notch and, after passing behind the hip joint, it descends in the posterior part of the thigh, dividing into two branches at the height of the popliteal fossa of the knee: the tibial and common peroneal nerves.

common peroneal nerve
The lateral branch of the two into which the sciatic nerve divides. It passes laterally behind the tibiofibular joint and borders the head of the fibula, passing to the anterolateral part of the leg. It bifurcates into two terminal branches: the superficial and deep peroneal nerves. In its short passage, the common peroneal nerve has articular branches that go to the knee joint and cutaneous branches to the skin of the region.

superficial peroneal nerve
The external branch of the common peroneal nerve, which follows a parallel path to the fibula, and sends muscular branches to the musculature of the region and cutaneous branches. Near the ankle joint, the superficial peroneal nerve bifurcates into the internal and external cutaneous dorsal nerves.

deep peroneal nerve
The medial branch of the common peroneal nerve. It traverses the leg vertically, in front of the tibia, and reaches the ankle joint to pass to the dorsal zone of the foot. It has branches to the anterior musculature of the leg, the ankle joint and the medial dorsal surface of the foot.

lateral dorsal cutaneous nerve
One of the terminal branches of the superficial fibular nerve. It runs down the external surface of the dorsal part of the foot and innervates the third, fourth and fifth toes.

medial dorsal cutaneous nerve
One of the terminal branches of the superficial fibular nerve that crosses the medial surface of the dorsal part of the foot, innervating the first and second toes.

tibial nerve
The medial branch of the sciatic nerve. It continues the path of the sciatic nerve and descends the leg behind the tibia. It has branches to the knee joint, the posterior musculature of the dorsal part of the leg and the skin of this region. When it reaches the ankle joint, it passes behind the medial malleolus and goes to the sole of the foot, where it divides into the medial and lateral plantar nerves. It also has a branch to the skin of the heel called the internal calcaneal nerve.

sural nerve
A nerve that originates from the tibial nerve and crosses the back of the leg superficially to reach the ankle, which it passes to reach the lateral border of the foot.

saphenous nerve
One of the branches of the femoral nerve which divides in the superior part of the thigh. It passes along the medial side of the thigh, the knee and the leg and crosses the ankle joint in front of the medial malleolus, to terminate in the medial border of the foot. It has branches to the skin of the medial face of the thigh, the knee, the leg and the foot.

lateral plantar nerve
After crossing behind the lateral malleolus, the tibial nerve reaches the sole of the foot and emits a lateral branch that innervates the musculature and skin of this area.

medial plantar nerve
When it reaches the sole of the foot, the tibial nerve emits a medial branch which innervates the musculature and skin of the area, and has digital nervous branches that go to the first, second and third toes.

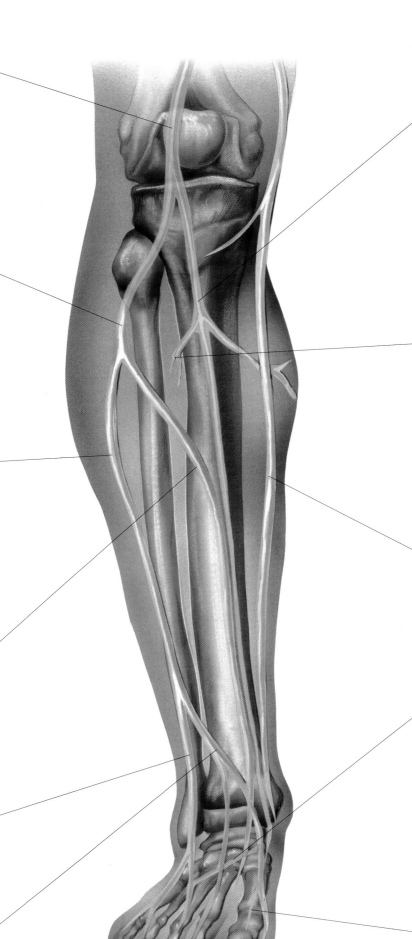

148

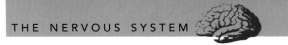

THE THIGH

lateral cutaneous nerve of the thigh
A nerve that originates from the first roots of the lumbosacral plexus. In the inferior extremity, it divides into an anterior or femoral branch and a posterior or gluteal branch, which innervate the superficial cutaneous zones of these regions.

femoral nerve
A thick nerve that originates in the lumbosacral plexus. It goes to the inferior extremity through the inguinal ligament and divides into four branches: the external and internal musculocutaneous nerves, the quadriceps nerve and the saphenous nerve.

obturator nerve
A nerve formed by the union of the anterior branches of the second, third and fourth lumbar spinal nerves. It descends to the pelvic cavity where it divides into different branches that go to the adductor muscles of the thigh.

nerve to sartorius
A branch of the femoral nerve that innervates the sartorius muscle and emits prolongations to the superficial area of the anterior face of the thigh, innervating the skin of this area.

vastus lateralis nerve
A branch of the femoral nerve that innervates the vastus lateralis muscle.

rectus femoris nerve
A branch of the femoral nerve that innervates the rectus femoris muscle.

sciatic nerve

inguinal ligament
A thin, fibrous ligament that extends obliquely from the anterosuperior iliac spine to the pubis. It marks the limit between the pelvic and femoral regions. The vessels and nerves that go to the inferior extremity pass under the inguinal ligament.

sciatic nerve
The largest nerve in the body. After its origin in the lumbosacral plexus it leaves the pelvis through the greater sciatic notch and passes behind the hip joint, arriving at the posterior part of the thigh by the gluteal region. It crosses the thigh from top to bottom, emitting branches for the muscles of that zone and, when it arrives at the level of the popliteal fossa of the knee, it is divided into two branches: the tibial and common peroneal nerves.

medial cutaneous branch of the femoral nerve
A branch of the femoral nerve that innervates some muscles of the superomedial part of the thigh and the skin that covers it.

saphenous nerve
One of the branches of the femoral nerve which descends along the medial side of the thigh and reaches the knee, sending branches to the skin and articulation of this area. It then divides into patellar and tibial branches.

vastus medialis nerve
A branch of the femoral nerve that innervates the vastus medialis muscle.

crural nerve
A branch of the femoral nerve that innervates the vastus intermedius muscle.

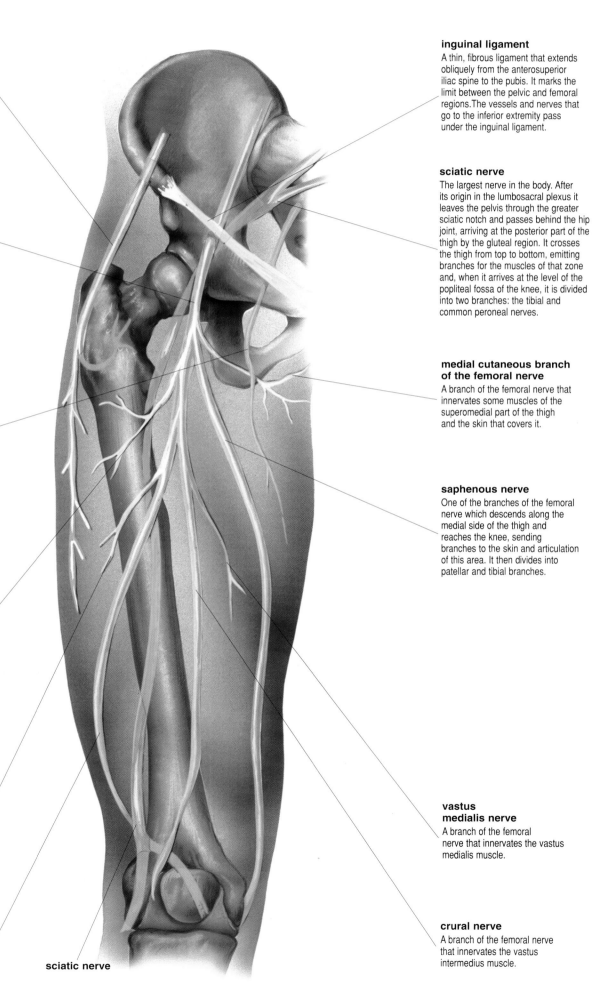

149

VISION. THE EYE

pupil
An orifice located in the centre of the iris, through which light penetrates to the eyeball. It is surrounded by a sphincter which causes its expansion (mydriasis) or contraction (miosis).

palpebral sulcus
The superior and inferior palpebral sulci are almost semicircular folds formed by the skin that covers the eyelid.

eyelids
Two cutaneous folds, one superior and the other inferior, that cover the anterior part of the eyeball. The orbicular muscles of the eyelids, which are located inside the eyelids, and the levator muscle of the eyelids located in the superior eyelid, ensure their mobility.

lacrimal canals
Thin ducts that originate in the lacrimal puncta, turn inwards and terminate in the lacrimal sac. Their function is to carry tears and any foreign bodies from the conjunctiva through the nasolacrimal groove and deliver them to the inferior meatus of the nasal cavity.

lacrimal glands
Grape-like clusters of glands located just inside the orbit, superior and lateral to the eyeball. They contain tiny secretory ducts which secrete the key ingredients and most of the volume of the tears which bathe the conjunctival surfaces and all the external surface of the eyeball.

lacrimal sac
A cylindrical cavity that receives the lacrimal canal and is continued downwards by the nasolacrimal duct.

lacrimal caruncle
Reddish or pink eminence located in the internal palpebral commissure.

eyelashes
Small hairs that line the free edges of the eyelids. They defend the eye against foreign bodies. Among them are the orifices of tiny sebaceous and sweat glands.

palpebral conjunctive tissue
The membrane or mucosa that covers the internal surface of the eyelids and extends backwards to cover the sclera.

iris
Ring-like pigmented tissue whose muscles control the amount of light entering the eye. The hole in the centre of the iris is the pupil. The iris is composed of smooth muscle innervated by autonomic nerves.

sclera
A layer of connective tissue that surrounds the eyeball, except anteriorly, where it is surrounded by the cornea. The sclera has a whitish colour and is not transparent.

lacrimal puncta
Two small orifices located above the lacrimal papillae, which are eminences located in the internal palpebral commissure.

nasolacrimal duct
A descending continuation of the lacrimal sac. It terminates in the nasal fossae, where the lacrimal secretions are delivered through the inferior meatus located under the inferior nasal concha.

FUNDUS OCULI
A representation of the surface of the retina as seen through the pupil using an ophthalmoscope.

retina
The retina is the internal layer of the eyeball and lines two thirds of it. It is formed of nervous tissue similar to that of the brain and contains cells that receive light and convert it into nervous impulses that are transmitted to the brain.

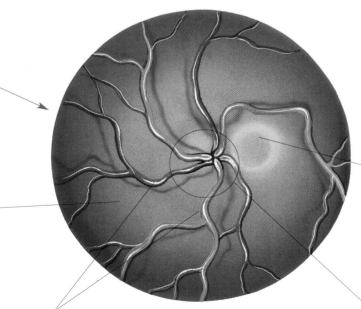

macula
Also known as the fovea centralis. A specialized area in the posterior of the retina, rich in photoreceptor cells, where the image is focused.

arteries and veins of the retina
The retinal artery and vein reach the interior of the eyeball through the papilla in parallel with the optic nerve. Inside the eye they branch out over the entire retinal surface.

papilla
A circular, yellowish-white area, located in the posterior region of the retina, where it joins the optical nerve and where the central arteries and veins of the retina terminate.

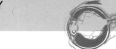

VISION. OCULAR MUSCULATURE

medial rectus muscle of the eye

A muscle that crosses the medial surface of the eyeball, from the common tendon of origin of the rectus muscles of the eye in the vertex of the ocular cavity. It is inserted in the ocular sclera, a few millimetres inside the medial border of the cornea. It turns the cornea outwards. The action of this muscle in one eye is synchronous with that of the lateral rectus muscle of the other eye.

superior rectus muscle of the eye

A thin muscle located below and parallel to the levator muscle of the superior eyelid. It originates posteriorly in a tendon that serves as the common origin of the four rectus muscles of the eye and is attached to the vertex of the orbit. The muscle extends over the eyeball and is inserted in the sclera, a few millimetres above the superior border of the cornea. When contracted it turns the cornea upwards and inwards, allowing the eye to move in this direction. Its contraction in one eye is coordinated with the inferior oblique muscle of the other eye.

superior oblique muscle of the eye

A muscle located in the roof of the orbit, internal to the levator muscle of the superior eyelid. It originates posteriorly to the levator muscle and goes to the medial border of the orbital foramen where it is converted into a tendon which is attached to a ligament that makes an acute angle, passes below the superolateral muscle of the eye and is inserted in the superior internal area of the sclera. It acts to turn the cornea downwards and outwards.

optical nerve

A thick nerve that enters the ocular cavity and penetrates the eyeball through its posterior face. The optical nerve sends the visual sensations received by the retina to the brain.

levator muscle of the superior eyelid

A flat, triangular muscle that crosses the vault of the orbital cavity from anterior to posterior. It originates in the bone forming the fundus of the orbit and is inserted in the subcutaneous tissue of the upper eyelid. It acts to elevate the superior eyelid.

151

orbicularis oculi muscle

A circular facial muscle that surrounds the palpebral orifice. It originates in the internal angle of the eye and is inserted in the external angle. It is attached to the skin of the eyelids in all its trajectory. Its action is to open or close the eyelid.

inferior rectus muscle of the eye

The inferior rectus muscle has a common posterior origin with the other rectus muscles of the eye. It crosses the floor of the ocular cavity and is inserted in the anterior inferior part of the sclera of the eyeball, a few millimetres below the inferior border of the cornea. Its contraction turns the cornea downwards and inwards, directing the vision in this direction. Its action in one eye is coordinated with the superior oblique muscle of the other eye.

inferior oblique muscle of the eye

A muscle that crosses the floor of the ocular cavity from its internal or nasal part towards the external part. It originates in the bone forming the floor of the orbit, crosses the inferior hemisphere of the eyeball below the inferior rectus muscle and is inserted into the inferior external area of the sclera. Its action is to turn the cornea upwards and outwards.

lateral rectus muscle of the eye

A muscle that crosses the lateral surface of the eyeball, from the tendon that is the common origin of the rectus muscles of the eye in the vertex of the ocular cavity, to the ocular sclera, a few millimetres outside the external edge of the cornea. Its action is to turn the cornea outwards when contracted. Its action is synchronous with that of the medial rectus muscle of the opposite eye, ensuring both eyes turn in the same direction.

VISION. THE EYEBALL

iris
A structure that forms part of the intermediate layer of the wall of the eyeball. It is disc-shaped and located in the anterior face of the eye. The hole in the centre of the iris is the pupil. It varies in colour according to its transparency and vascularization, determining the colour of the eyes.

ciliary body
An internal protuberance located between the iris and the choroidea, that contains the ciliary muscle and the ciliary processes, which are formed by a dense vascular network and secrete the vitreous humour. Its cross-section is triangular and its shape is annular, surrounding the iris externally.

suspensory ligament of the lens
Transparent fibres that unite the internal edge of the ciliary body with the periphery of the crystalline lens, maintaining it fixed in its position.

vitreous body
A viscous, transparent fluid that fills all the ocular cavity located behind the crystalline lens.

sclera
A layer of connective tissue that surrounds the eyeball, except anteriorly, where it is surrounded by the cornea. The sclera has a whitish colour and is not transparent.

cornea
A layer of connective tissue that covers the anterior part of the eyeball, causing it to protrude. The cornea is totally transparent, in order to let light pass.

choroid
The intermediate layer of the three which form the wall of the eyeball, the choroidea is formed by a complex network of blood vessels that nourish the retina. It surrounds two-thirds of the eyeball, the rest being covered by the iris.

retina
The retina is the internal layer of the eyeball and lines two-thirds of it. It is formed of nervous tissue similar to that of the brain, and contains cells that receive light and convert it into nervous impulses that are transmitted to the brain.

papilla
A circular, yellowish-white area, located in the posterior region of the retina, where it joins the optical nerve and where the central arteries and veins of the retina terminate.

152

anterior chamber
The space between the cornea and the iris, which is occupied by vitreous humour.

pupil
An orifice located in the centre of the iris, through which light penetrates to the eyeball. It is surrounded by a sphincter that causes its expansion (mydriasis) or contraction (miosis).

posterior chamber
A space located behind the iris and in front of the crystalline lens. It contains vitreous humour.

crystalline lens
An epithelial structure located behind the iris. Its anterior surface is bathed by vitreous humour and the posterior face by the vitreous body. It functions as a biconvex lens whose changes of shape allow light impulses to be focused on the retina.

central artery and vein of the retina
Two blood vessels that reach the retina following the axis of the optic nerve and terminate in the interior of the eyeball at the papilla, forming branches that cover the retinal surface.

optical nerve
A thick nerve that unites the eyeball with the central nervous system, transporting the light sensations, converted in the retina into nervous stimuli, to the brain, specifically to the area of the occipital cerebral cortex in charge to perceive consciously these sensations.

VISION. CONSTITUTION OF THE RETINA

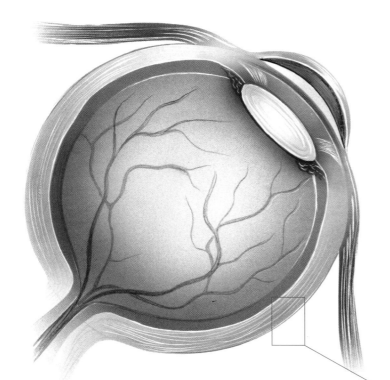

RETINA

The retina is the internal layer of the eyeball and lines two-thirds of it. It is formed of nervous tissue similar to that of the brain and contains cells that receive light and convert it into nervous impulses that are transmitted to the brain. In the posterior zone of the retina there is an area containing many photoreceptor cells called the maculae, which give clarity to the vision.

pigmentary epithelium
A layer of cells that produce a pigment called melanin, which protects and isolates the photoreceptor cells.

amacrine cells
Cells that associate and connect the bipolar cells and the ganglion cells, transmitting information about the light impulses received from one point of the retina to another.

photoreceptor cells
The photoreceptor cells are light-sensitive retinal cells (cones and rods), located below the pigmented epithelium. They contain chemicals called photopsin and rhodopsin which react to specific light wavelengths and trigger nerve impulses.

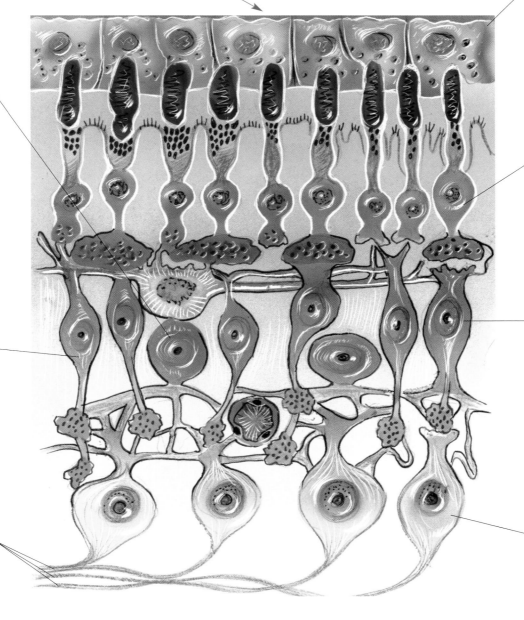

horizontal cells
Cells that fix the connections between the photoreceptors and the bipolar cells, transmitting information from the light impulses that are received in each point of the retina. Together with the amacrine cells they are called association cells.

bipolar cells
Cells connected by a synaptic union with the photoreceptors. They capture the nervous impulses generated by the photoreceptor cells and transport them to the ganglion cells.

optical nerve
The optical nerve is formed by the axons of the ganglion cells. It extends to the optical chiasm and, after the two optical nerves join, it goes to the optical thalamus and posteriorly to the occipital cerebral cortex or visual cortex.

ganglion cells
Nervous cells that receive the impulses transmitted by the bipolar cells and carry them to the brain through a long axon which becomes part of the optic nerve.

HEARING

pinna
The external, visible part of the ear, which surrounds the outer ear canal. It is composed principally of four cartilaginous structures called the helix, antihelix, tragus and antitragus.

helix
The curled rim of the outer part of the ear.

antihelix
Part of the cartilage of the ear which forms a curved elevation within or in front of the helix.

tympanic part of the temporal one
One of the parts of the temporal bone, whose horizontal area constitutes the roof of the external acoustic duct.

tympanic membrane or **eardrum**
A fibrous, elastic membrane that separates the external acoustic duct from the middle ear. Through its vibrations, sounds from the exterior are transmitted to the articulated ossicles of the tympanic cavity.

articulated ossicles
Three articulated bones (malleus, incus and stapes) which transmit the vibrations of the tympanic membrane to the labyrinth.

semicircular ducts
Three tubes arranged in three different planes which have receptors that capture the movements of the endolymph. They are essential for the maintenance of posture and balance.

internal acoustic meatus
A bony duct located in the petrous bone. It gives passage to the vestibulocochlear and facial nerves and the intermediate nerve of Wrisberg, and connects the cochlea with the interior of the cranial cavity.

cochlea
A spiral duct located below the vestibule. It contains the organ of Corti, which transforms auditory sensations into nervous stimuli.

vestibule
An elongated cavity containing the articulated ossicles that communicates with the tympanic cavity through an orifice called the oval window.

154

external acoustic duct
Duct that communicates the pinna with the eardrum. It is covered by a prolongation of the skin of the pinna which is covered by very fine hairs.

facial nerve
A sensory motor nerve also known as the seventh cranial nerve which, after penetrating the internal acoustic duct, crosses the petrous bone by the Fallopian aqueduct and leaves the cranium through the stylomastoid foramen and divides into temporal and cervical terminal branches.

tympanic cavity
A cavity contained by the petrous segment of the temporal bone which houses the articulated ossicles. It corresponds to the part of the auditory system called the middle ear.

internal jugular vein
The internal jugular vein originates in the union of the cranial venous sinus in the area of the petrous bone, and receives the venous blood coming from the intracranial structures.

Eustachian tube
A duct that connects the tympanic cavity with the pharynx and permits air from the nasal fossas to reach the cavities of the ear, thereby balancing the pressure on both sides of the eardrum.

peristaphyline muscle
A muscle that is inserted in the petrous bone and the proximities of the Eustachian tube and extends to the soft palate, which it tenses when contracted.

labyrinth
A set of osseous cavities located in the sinus of the petrous bone, which correspond to the internal ear and contain membranous structures filled with a fluid called endolymph. There are three cavities which form the labyrinth: the cochlea, vestibule and semicircular canals.

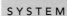

OLFACTION

nasal vestibule
A widening that constitutes the initial part of both nasal fossae. The vestibule, like the rest of the nasal fossae, is covered by a mucosa rich in mucous glands and small hairs that filter the air.

concha
A bony protuberance covered by nasal mucosa located in the lateral walls of the nasal fossae. Its function is to create turbulence in the inspired air, thus warming and humidifying it before it reaches the pharynx.

olfactory bulb

olfactory nerve
Also called the first cranial nerve. The olfactory nerve is formed by the axons of nervous cells that cross the cribiform lamina of the ethmoid bone from the olfactory mucosa in the nasal fossas and terminate in the olfactory bulb.

olfactory tract
A cord of nervous tissue that transmits the olfactory sensations captured by the nasal fossas to the cerebral centres which interpret them.

sphenoidal sinus
A cavity located in the sphenoid bone, which communicates with the nasal fossas through orifices located behind the conchae. Its function is to warm the air before it reaches the inferior respiratory tract.

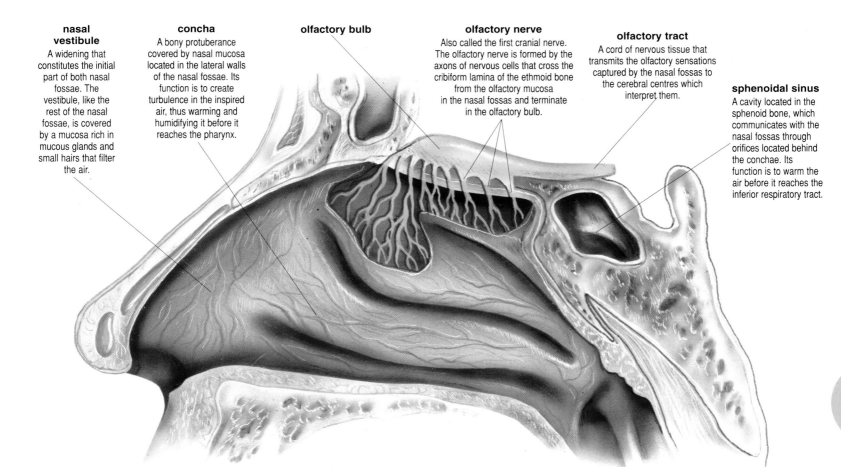

olfactory glomerulus
The point where the olfactory nerves are united with the mitral cells, whose axons extend along the olfactory bulb and constitute the nerve fibres of the olfactory tract.

nerve fibres of the olfactory tract
The nervous cells of the olfactory bulb, called mitral cells, are united, on the one hand, with the olfactory nerves and, on the other hand, emit prolongations or axons that carry the olfactory sensations through the olfactory tract to the brain.

olfactory bulb
A swelling located at the end of the olfactory tract, over the cribiform lamina of the ethmoid bone. The nervous fibres that make up the olfactory nerves reach the olfactory bulb and are transmitted to the brain in the area of the hippocampus.

cribiform lamina
A part of the ethmoid bone located between the cranial cavity and the nasal fossas. It has a series of small orifices that allow the passage of branches of the olfactory nerve.

olfactory mucosa
Mucosa that covers the posterior superior part of the nasal fossae and contains the nervous cells specialized in capturing smells.

olfactory gland
Multiple glands which are dispersed between the olfactory cells of the nasal mucosa and which produce a mucous secretion.

olfactory cells
Nerve cells specialized in capturing smells. The olfactory cells are bipolar cells that emit a series of small cilia at one extreme which go to the nasal cavity, and at the other extreme they continue as nervous prolongations or axons, to form the olfactory nerve.

GUSTATION. TONGUE

LINGUAL PAPILLAE
Small papillae that cover the surface of the buccal mucosa and contain the taste buds. They can be of different types, according to their shape and function.

■ area of bitter taste sensation

■ area of sour taste sensation

■ area of salt taste sensation

■ area of sweet taste sensation

terminal sulcus
A V-shaped sulcus that crosses the tongue transversally and delimits the posterior aspect of the tongue, which then descends vertically to form the lingual tonsils.

fungiform papillae
The fungiform papillae are distributed along the edges of the tongue and are bigger than the filiform papillae. They contain taste buds located in the superior surface of the lingual papillae.

filiform papillae
The filiform papillae are simple elevations of the epithelium of the buccal mucosa, which constitute the smallest type of taste buds. They are very numerous and are distributed over the two anterior thirds of the tongue's surface.

circumvallate papillae
The large, prominent bumps on the top surface of the back of the tongue are a fourth type of papilla called circumvallate papillae. They are located along the circumvallate line and contain taste buds that allow the back of the tongue to distinguish sour and bitter tastes.

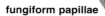

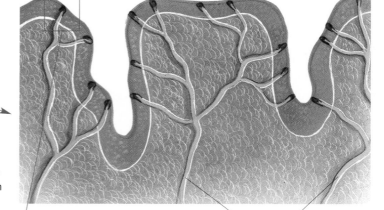

nerve fibres
Fibres emitted from each taste bud which transmit the nervous stimuli generated by the taste receptors by means of different nerves which go to the brain, specifically to an area of the cerebral cortex called the limen insula.

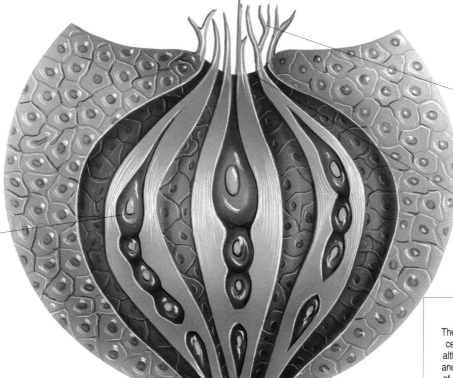

microvilli
Tiny villi or taste hairs that line the outside of the gustatory cells. They show through the gustatory pore and they provide the receptor surface necessary to capture flavours.

gustatory cells
Each taste bud contains around twenty gustatory cells whose function is to capture taste. They are stimulated by the substances responsible for a specific taste, which are dissolved in the saliva, and turn this sensation into a nervous stimulus.

gustatory pore
An orifice in the epithelium that lines the buccal mucosa and communicates it with the cells located in the interior of the taste bud.

TASTE BUD
The taste buds, containing the gustatory cells, are mainly located in the tongue although they also cover the soft palate and the pharynx. They capture the taste of any substance ingested and transmit the information to the brain through the nervous fibres.

156

TOUCH. TACTILE CORPUSCLES

free nerve endings
Tiny nervous terminations that penetrate to the superficial layers of the dermis. Although they have no specialized functions, they capture sensation of light touch, pressure, pain and temperature.

Meissner's corpuscle
Encapsulated terminations of sensitive nerve fibres located in the superficial part of the dermis that capture smooth tactile stimuli, such as rubbing. Meissner's corpuscles are distributed over all the skin, but are especially abundant in the finger tips.

Pacinian corpuscle
Encapsulated nervous terminations located in deep zones of the dermis. Pacinian corpuscles are specialized in capturing feelings of deep pressure and vibrations and probably play an important role in the perception of movement.

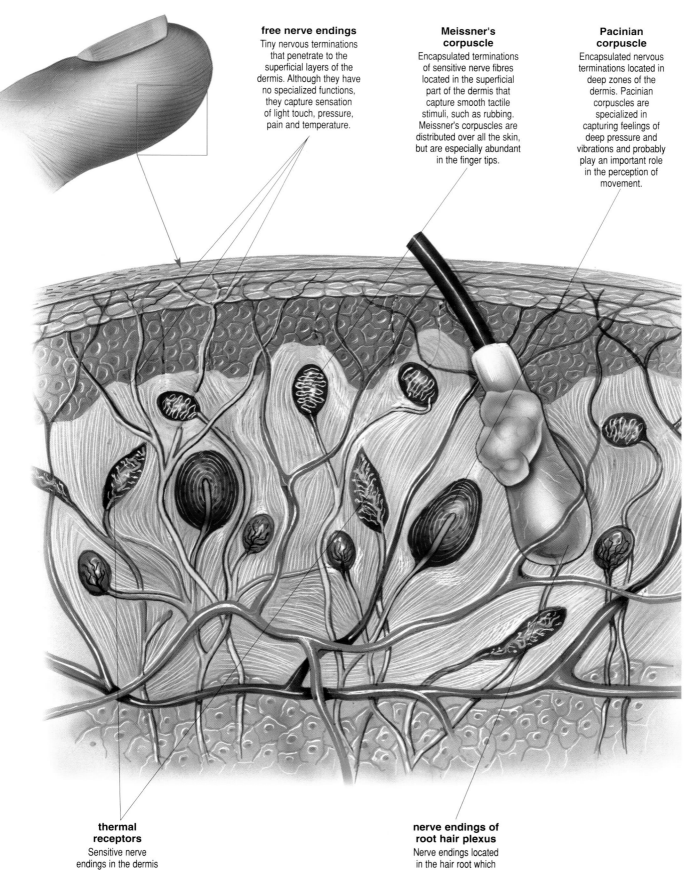

epidermis
The superficial, external layer of the skin, formed by layers of cells that are constantly renovated, with the dead keratinized cells flaking off to be replaced by others.

157

dermis
The intermediate of the three skin layers. Composed of loose connective tissue and fibrous tissue, it contains many nerve terminations responsible for capturing tactile sensations.

hypodermis
The deepest layer of the skin, located below the dermis. It is formed of loose connective tissue and contains abundant adipose tissue, which acts as a cushion for the organs below (muscles, bones, viscera, etc.).

thermal receptors
Sensitive nerve endings in the dermis specialized in capturing thermal sensations such as cold and heat.

nerve endings of root hair plexus
Nerve endings located in the hair root which capture any sensation experienced by the external part of the hair.

INDEX